EMPOWERED!

A Parent's Survival Guide to Navigating the
Mental Healthcare System

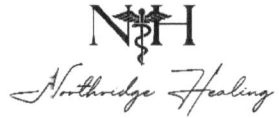

Stephanie M. Macke, DO

EMPOWERED! A Parent's Survival Guide to Navigating the Mental Healthcare System

Copyright © 2022 by Stephanie Macke

Cover Design by Dee Dee Book Covers

ISBNs:
979-8-9866081-2-9 (hardcover)
979-8-9866081-0-5 (paperback)
979-8-9866081-1-2 (eBook)

Published by:

N♱H
Northridge Healing

Burning Soul Press

DEDICATION

To God, I devote myself.
May You use this book to bring comfort
to those who feel lost.

To my husband, Steven.
Your love and support have given me so much strength.
Thank you for being my partner in all things. I love you.

To my children (Brooklyn, Athena, Alexander,
Tyler, and Hunter).
I am here for you always.

To the moms and dads who feel overwhelmed.
You are not alone.

CONTENTS

INTRODUCTION

I am a parent. I am a physician. I am a utilizer of the mental health system. I am constantly amazed at the lack of resources readily available in mental health. If a 15-year-old male with new onset weight loss, loose stools, and abdominal pain presents to my medical office, I can obtain laboratory work (generally blood testing and stool cultures). If the patient needs specialist consultation based on the initial work up, I can call a pediatric gastroenterologist and have them seen within a week or two, sooner if the presentation is more severe. If, however, a 15-year-old male with depression leading to school absences, lack of close relationships, and reduced motivation in accomplishing daily activities presents to my medical office and needs counseling or more specialized medication management, sadly, it may take several months before a spot opens for the adolescent to be seen by a behavioral health provider.

When I decided on a career in medicine, I was immediately drawn to family practice. I was attracted to the idea of caring for parents and their children, and in some cases, their children's children, their nieces and nephews, their co-workers, and their friends. I enjoy the diversity of healthcare I face each day. In any one shift I may perform a skin biopsy, care for a newborn baby, treat diabetes, or help an elderly patient get in-home resources to maintain their independence. I appreciate integrative medicine and have adapted manual therapy, acupuncture, and supplementation into my medical recommendations. By far, the most common thing I have come to treat in primary care over the past decade is mental health.

Health is more than blood pressures, heart rates, weights, and oxygen saturations. In fact, there are four aspects to an individual's health: the physical, the psychological, the social and the spiritual. The field of mental health is unique in that it requires balance in all four categories. The cardiologist mostly worries about the heart. The urologist is most concerned about the bladder and kidneys. The pulmonologist primarily analyzes the lungs. The behavioral health provider must evaluate the physiology and anatomy of several organs whose ill behavior can mimic a mental health condition. While the behavioral specialist works through the physical characteristics of an individual, they must also become familiar with the individual's family genetics, social and physical environments, and spiritual connections. As you can see, there is a significant amount of information each behavioral health provider must review for every individual. Unfortunately, there are also not enough providers currently to meet the demand of those seeking services.

As a primary care provider, I am often the first person that sees a child for mental health concerns. This is especially true if the child is not yet of school age. Parents often appear as anxious as their child when they first visit my office. They are not sure if their child's behavior is a psychiatric condition, or if their child is just an "odd kid." Most adolescents will demonstrate at least some abnormal behaviors. When behaviors grow to the point they are significantly interfering with daily activities, last greater than four weeks, or are not age appropriate, further evaluation may be necessary (Bratten, 2011). Common concerns that are brought to physicians by parents include: not meeting developmental milestones, increased temper tantrums, difficulty with following directions, cannot learn to read or write and homework is taking several hours, lack of focus, extreme fearfulness, and frequent sadness (Bratten, 2011). It's not typically one behavior, or one incident, that causes the parent to schedule an appointment. Parents typically report increased frequency and intensity of concerning behaviors and are at a loss for appropriate resources available to assist their child in their journey to becoming a strong and well-adjusted adult.

Too often I see providers take a "one size fits all approach." They mean well, but often fail to emphasize the brain and body connection. Many problematic behaviors reflect how a child's autonomic state perceives and responds to stress. In *Empowered! A Parent's Survival Guide to Navigating the Mental Healthcare System*, I use over a decade of medical practice, as well as my own experience as a parent with children who suffer emotional regulation, to support your journey raising a child who struggles with mental health ailments. Please note that within the text I use many examples of patients I have treated to help you connect with the material. For privacy reasons, names and other identifying characteristics have been changed.

This book is not meant to be a replacement for medical advice, diagnosis, or treatment from your child's healthcare team. These chapters are meant to provide educational support along your child's journey by connecting the dots in a complex system. If you feel your child is exhibiting concerning behaviors, I strongly recommend requesting an evaluation through a qualified medical provider. It is important to consult your child's providers before using any information, ideas, or products discussed within this book. In addition, as a parent, if you feel your own mental health is fragile, it's important to seek opportunities for self-care. You will not be able to fully support your child if you are struggling as well. Like the flight attendants say, "Put on your own oxygen mask first, then help those around you."

The mental health world is one of the most challenging ones I have found to navigate. I often wonder why if a good psychological state is so crucial to physical health, social relationships, work productivity, and overall mental wellbeing it is the most daunting field to find assistance. My children have waited several months for an appointment with a provider for therapy or medication management. I am often frustrated by the lack of continuity between the inpatient and outpatient worlds. I see the lack of resources available to my patients. There appears to be minimal education to parents regarding care from their child's diagnoses through a full treatment plan. There is less information presented on how best to add the child's school to the treatment team. My hope in writing this book is to provide parents with tools they need to feel comfortable navigating the mental health system. While every effort has been made to ensure the accuracy of the information presented, neither the author nor the publisher assumes any responsibility for errors.

Chapter 1

YOU ARE NOT ALONE ON YOUR JOURNEY

<u>*Ryan's Story*</u>

"9-1-1, what's your emergency?"

Silence.

Ryan's mother sat on the bathroom floor; her back pressed up to the closed door. She drew her legs into her chest and stared at the cell phone in her right hand. Words could not leave her lips. She had been crying for the past hour. She knew what she needed to do, yet her fingers trembled as she made the urgent call. She tried to pull herself together to respond to the operator.

"Hello, 9-1-1, is anyone there?" the operator asked.

"Hello. I am requesting the assistance of the Crisis Intervention Team at my home," she finally declared. "My ten-year-old son is currently exhibiting physical violence and refusing to get into our vehicle. I need help in getting him transported to the stress center for a psychiatric evaluation."

It was October. Night had crept in. The temperature was cool, but not cold. It had been raining and the damp smell circulated within the air. The evening had begun a couple of hours earlier with ten-year-old Ryan watching television with his older brother. For a while, the two boys had been getting along. They both enjoyed the same YouTubers and catching up on the latest postings while finishing their burritos from dinner seemed like an idea they could equally buy into. Within twenty minutes, the two boys started to bicker. Ryan was trying to watch Mark Rober's new Glitter Bomb segment while his brother, having already watched the episode a dozen times, was telegraphing the upcoming dialogue. It didn't take long for Ryan to become annoyed by his brother's actions.

"Stop saying what he's saying Jonathan!" Ryan yelled at him. Jonathan looked towards his brother. He could see Ryan's frustration. For whatever reason, it brought Jonathan joy knowing his brother was aggravated, so Jonathan continued his behavior. Ryan got up from his spot on the sofa, walked towards his sibling sitting in a nearby chair and punched him in the arm. His older sibling was a half size bigger than he was, but Ryan didn't care. Jonathan punched him back. Ryan's emotions heightened.

"Both of you go to your rooms and calm down," their mother told them. She had entered the living room when she overheard the children's rising voices.

"He started it!" Jonathan whined. "Why should I have to be punished for what he did?"

Ryan kept his eyes on his brother, and again entering his brother's personal space, slugged hard into his shoulder.

"Ow!" Jonathan cried. "See?"

"Boys, go up to your rooms. We'll talk about this in a few minutes." Their mother had hoped separating the children would get them to cool off and then she could talk to them individually about the incident. While she could easily have stepped between the two boys when they were younger, as they had been growing their mere size meant she could be significantly injured if she came between their blows.

"No." One word. No more. That's all Ryan said. His tone was flat and assertive. His eyes appeared as though they could have borne a hole through his brother's soul. Jonathan stood up and headed to the staircase towards his room. Ryan followed him and moved further into Jonathan's space. He managed to get in front of Jonathan on the staircase and held one arm to the wall and the other to the banister. He took a strong stance and barricaded anyone from getting to the second floor.

"Let me up the stairs Ryan!" Jonathan shouted as he tried to move his brother out of the way. He pushed his brother's arm down and, having the advantage of being physically larger squeezed between his brother and the wall making his way to his room. Ryan again followed. As Jonathan tried desperately to get into his bedroom and close the door, Ryan ran into Jonathan's room.

"Get out!" Jonathan screamed.

"No," Ryan replied, again with the flat, usual tone.

The boy's mother called for her spouse who had been sitting in a separate room. When Ryan started his meltdowns, they could last a few minutes to a few hours, but typically they were physically aggressive. The boy's parents headed upstairs after them. While they were able to redirect Ryan from Jonathan, it unfortunately ended in Ryan's wrath being transferred to them. Ryan became violent. He took both of his arms and slammed into his mother, pushing her into the wall. He started to kick his father. He may have been a youngster, but he was already nearly five feet tall and weighed 125lbs. His father restrained Ryan to avoid causing harm to anyone else, including Ryan himself. Ryan bit his father and blood came to the surface. It was clear Ryan's behavior was escalating. Ryan's parents tried to keep him out of the way of the other children in the home. While doing so, they both continued to sustain punches, kicks, pushes, and even had a few objects thrown at them.

During this event, Ryan's mother recalled a conversation she had with another child's mother. The other child was a nine-year-old boy who suffered from an inability to emotionally regulate. The boy's mother had explained that her son, Benjamin, had become increasingly agitated at school. Benjamin had been meeting with school counselors, had an individualized educational plan (IEP), yet the teachers were not equipped to handle Benjamin's needs. There was no known trigger for Benjamin's behavioral issues at school. One Wednesday afternoon, during what appeared to be out of the blue, Benjamin got angry with his teacher and hit her. After talking with Benjamin's counselor, it had been advised that he be evaluated through the local crisis center for possible inpatient evaluation based on his past psychological concerns and the new change in his functional state.

Ryan suffered from anxiety and depression. At least anxiety and depression were the diagnoses provided by a clinical psychologist on a recent evaluation. Ryan's parents had been concerned about his continued aggressive behavior despite therapeutic intervention. They scheduled an appointment with the clinic to have him assessed. Based on the results of Ryan's testing, he participated in weekly therapy targeted towards learning coping skills. When this did not appear to be enough and the emotional outbursts continued, his pediatrician started him on a medication, Zoloft (sertraline), for mood regulation. Unfortunately, even the combination of therapy and medication management were not as successful as his parents desired. Ryan's behavior had slowly progressed to a dangerous new level. He was becoming a physical threat not just to his parents, but to the other children in the home.

Ryan's mother asked him to follow her to the car. She told him they were going to talk to a doctor to help him calm down. Her intentions were to drive him to the crisis center for an evaluation, like what Benjamin had recently gone through. Despite several requests, Ryan refused to head to the vehicle. Ryan's father stayed with him in an effort to keep Ryan from causing harm to his siblings, while his mother left the scene to make the 911 call.

Ten minutes after the urgent request for assistance, two male police officers arrived at the home. Walking to meet the men in the driveway, Ryan's mother started the conversation and said, "Hello officers. My son, Ryan, is ten years old. He struggles with anxiety and depression. Occasionally when Ryan is overwhelmed, he gets very physically violent. Ryan and his brother had an altercation tonight and this has flared up Ryan. The other children in the home are safe, but I need to take Ryan to the stress center for an evaluation. Something isn't right with Ryan tonight. He's more aggressive than usual. I called to ask for assistance to help transport Ryan to the facility as he is resisting us." Her voice was clear yet frazzled. She hadn't wanted the family's night to turn out like this. She was worried about what would happen when they got to the hospital's stress center for the evaluation. Did this mean she was a bad parent? Was Ryan going to be a terrible teenager and eventually adult that hurt others when he lost his temper? Was there more to the puzzle than anxiety and depression? Had the psychologist missed something during the evaluation? Many questions raced through her mind in those minutes, and the many hours that were to come. Most of the thoughts were not helpful in the moment and only increased her own anxiety further. She tried to remain calm, and she had decided Ryan needed to see a strong front, even if she felt out of control herself.

Ryan ran down the stairs and looked out the window only to see his mother speaking with the officers. It had not been until this point he had realized his parents were serious about getting him evaluated. Ryan immediately stopped protesting. He couldn't believe they would call the police on him. He put on his sneakers and walked through the kitchen and out the garage door. Ryan proceeded to get into the backseat of the car. He did not say a word.

Ryan's father walked out of the home behind him. He had not left Ryan's side for some time. As he walked out of the home he was met by the taller, thinner, of the two officers. "Do you think he has relaxed enough to be able to travel safely?" the officer asked Ryan's father.

"He only stopped being aggressive once he saw your vehicle in the driveway," Ryan's father replied. "I am okay attempting to drive him to the hospital now that he's in the car, but I'm not sure what to do if he tries to jump out of the vehicle while we are driving. I wouldn't put that response past him." The police officer opened the backdoor of the car and demonstrated to Ryan's father how to "lock" the door so that it could not be opened except from the outside.

While the officer spoke to Ryan's father, his partner opened the opposing backseat door and started to talk to Ryan. "Are you Ryan?"

"Yes," Ryan said matter of fact.

"I hear you're having a tough night," the officer replied.

Ryan nodded.

"Well, your parents are concerned, and they are going to take you to a doctor so you can feel better. Do you think you can go with them?"

Ryan nodded again.

The officer backed up and Ryan's mother moved into the backseat alongside her son. Ryan's father moved back to the front of the vehicle, secured his seatbelt, and prepared to drive.

Ryan whispered to his mother, "Mom, he has a gun. I can't believe you called the cops, and they brought a gun!" She didn't respond. She didn't know how to answer his comment.

"If he has more issues during your drive, please call us back and we'll take him in the back of our vehicle," the first officer said. He spoke in a loud, clear voice so Ryan could overhear his comment.

For the most part, the ride was quiet. Ryan's question broke the silence. "What's going to happen when we get there?" His voice did not change in intonation but was softer than when he had been at home.

"I don't know," his mother stated.

"Will I get to go back home?" Ryan asked.

"I don't know," she said again. The truth was, she didn't know. What happens when a child is violent and desiring to hurt others without a single care as to the consequence? She was certain this behavior was not ordinary. She had four older children at home that never seemed to have this type of struggle.

When they arrived at the stress center Ryan's father pulled the vehicle up to the front door and assisted Ryan and his mother out of the car. Ryan and his mother walked to the sliding glass doors and entered the building while his father parked the car. It was late. By now it was half past ten. The facility was empty except for a woman sitting behind a large desk. Her hair was braided back behind her head, and she wore large glasses and an oversized white sweater. She looked up from what she was doing and gazed towards the two visitors. "May I help you?"

"Yes. This is Ryan. We are here for him to be evaluated. He's having a rough night." his mother explained.

"Has he been here before?" the woman asked.

"No," Ryan's mother replied, still trying to keep her composure.

"Please complete these forms," the receptionist stated as she handed Ryan's mother a clipboard with several printed sheets. "I'll also need a driver's license and an insurance card."

Ryan's mother completed the documents. Her husband entered the building and joined her and Ryan. He sat down in the chair beside Ryan placing Ryan between his parents. The receptionist looked over her desk, "If you are all done with those, I can take them." Ryan's mother stood up, walked to the desk, and handed her the borrowed clipboard. "The triage nurse will be with you in a few moments," the woman said as she collected the paperwork.

The stress center was cold. It maintained the sterile smell that comes with being in a hospital. Many of the lights were shut off due to being evening hours and the only lights on were bright fluorescents. The custodial staff were moving about cleaning trash cans and mopping floors, their chores generating the only sounds to echo the halls. Ryan sat still in his seat. His eyes remained fixated on his sneakers. He was wearing an oversized hooded sweatshirt. The hood was up over his head and his hands were shoved in the front pocket. He didn't make a sound.

After twenty minutes or so, a younger woman came to the waiting room. She wore a blue t-shirt with the facility's logo, lighter blue scrub pants and colorful Dansko clogs. Her blonde hair was pulled back in a ponytail. Her name badge listed "RN," registered nurse. She appeared much more awake than Ryan and his parents. "Ryan? Are you ready to come back with me?"

Ryan looked up in the direction of the woman. His mother could tell his initial response was to say no, but he was aware he didn't really have an option. He stood up and slowly followed her through the thick double doors. Ryan's parents followed him, and the doors clicked together as they locked behind them. The nurse led the family to the second room on the right. It was a small private room where she could ask additional questions. Four wooden chairs with leather seats sat in a circle in the center of the room. Ryan tried to push one back but struggled with its weight. His mother looked around the room. The walls contained no artwork and showed only their dingy white color. The nurse rolled in a portable computer desk to complete her documentation. On top of the computer's keyboard was a "patient belongings" plastic bag.

"I'll need your shoes, anything in your pockets, and the string from your sweatshirt hood," she declared while making eye contact with Ryan. Ryan took off his shoes and handed them to her.

"Why are you taking my shoes?" he asked.

"So you don't throw them at me," she said calmly. "You can use these instead." The nurse reached from atop her portable computer desk and grabbed a pair of socks with rubber tread. The socks would help Ryan not to slip on the floor while he walked on the cold tile. He removed his personal socks and placed the facility foot coverings on his feet. The nurse collected his items and placed them in the large item collection bag. "And the string from your sweatshirt?"

He looked at her quizzically. "So you don't strangle yourself or someone else," his mother explained. He looked at her with an expression of, "Are you kidding me?" but pulled the string out of his hoodie nonetheless. The nurse placed the string in the bag. Her last action was to place Ryan's medical identification bracelet on his wrist.

The nurse moved on to the interview portion of the intake and proceeded to ask questions about Ryan's medical history. She asked about previous diagnoses, surgeries, medications, allergies, and family history. The nurse asked Ryan whether he felt he was going to hurt himself or someone else to which he promptly responded, "No." When the healthcare worker had checked all the boxes for her intake review, she notified Ryan's parents that the medical provider would be in to evaluate Ryan shortly.

It was a Licensed Clinical Social Worker (LCSW) that came in next to get the history of the night's episode. Ryan, his father, and his mother spent the greater part of an hour recounting the events of the day, Ryan's past medical history and discussing Ryan's experience with his counselor and pediatrician for mental health services. Sometimes the questions from the LCSW included the three of them. A portion, however, was conducted with Ryan's parents separate from him. After the LCSW believed she had obtained all the necessary information to make a reasonable call for admission to the inpatient facility she stated, "Thank you for providing me with these details. I am going to speak with the psychiatrist on call and I will be back shortly to let you know what he decides." The LCSW left the room.

Ryan sat in the heavy wooden chair. He drew his legs into his chest and pulled his sweatshirt down over his knees. Ryan's parents worked hard to keep their eyes open. It was now nearing the early hours of the next day. As the clock made its way to nearly two in the morning the LCSW returned. "I had an opportunity to talk to the psychiatrist on call.

I told him that Ryan says he is not a threat to himself at this time and I explained how Ryan has been calm throughout the intake process. The doctor is aware of your concerns and knows Ryan has a counselor and that his pediatrician is prescribing Ryan's medication for anxiety. Our facility doesn't really provide inpatient care for Ryan's age group and so we are going to recommend he follow up in the next few days with his counselor and pediatrician," she said. She then proceeded to give Ryan his hoodie string and shoes back. "Do you have any questions?" the LCSW said in a voice that made his mother think she only asked because it was part of the discharge requirements.

Ryan's parents had a great deal of questions. Ryan had been aggressive, and this wasn't the first time. How do they handle this at home? Ryan's medication doesn't cover his meltdowns, why can't he be given something else? Are anxiety and depression the right diagnoses for Ryan? Why didn't the hospital say they didn't provide services for Ryan's age group hours ago when they were checking him in for an evaluation? It seemed as though the LCSW had done her job and those questions were not going to be answered on this night. Ryan's parents packed him up and drove him home. Ryan slept the entire thirty-minute drive. The next morning when he awoke in his bed, he was ready for breakfast and in a chipper mood. It was as though the past evening's events had not been acknowledged by Ryan at all. His parents, on the other hand, were exhausted and feeling overwhelmingly defeated. What was the next step in seeking help for Ryan?

Michelle's Story

Michelle recently celebrated her 15th birthday. It was spring, the sun was shining, and she was singing the latest High School Musical soundtrack. Michelle was an officer in the theater club at school and active in show choir. She maintained straight As despite taking the top honors classes. She was well liked by her teachers and had a close friend group she was able to confide in. Michelle's father and mother had divorced during her seventh-grade year. She had not been surprised when she heard the news. She had seen the writing on the wall.

Nevertheless, when they finally separated and she found herself bouncing between homes, she discovered the inconsistencies between residencies extremely challenging. In an effort to cope, she placed a great deal of effort into the things she could control: her appearance, her role in the drama department, and her academic merits.

Michelle struggled with anxiety. While she thrived in the high ability program, she put a lot of pressure on herself to be perfect. If Michelle missed a question on a test, she was devastated. Michelle cried when she had a wrong answer. She found her identity in perfection and an incorrect answer made her feel like less of a person. She argued her grade with her teacher, trying to get them to change their mind about the test result. Eventually her restlessness and feelings of inadequacy got the best of her, and Michelle shut down, unable to complete any other course work for the remaining day.

Michelle walked home after school, her eyes looking down to the sidewalk in front of her. She hid in her room. When her mother asked her how her day was, she screamed "Everyone hates me! I hate school! I'm never going back!" Michelle went on to complain that her stomach hurt. She didn't want to eat dinner. She hugged her teddy bear, buried her head in her pillow and cried herself to sleep. At first this occurred once a week, but as the school year progressed, the frequency increased.

Unfortunately for Michelle, her genetics came with a strong history of behavioral health ailments. When Michelle started to show signs of anxiety, her mother scheduled an appointment with a local therapist. Her mother had hoped therapy would teach Michelle ways to reduce her over-excited response to daily triggers. Michelle worked with the counselor on coping skills for six weeks before claiming, "I've got this!" and not wanting to return to see her therapist.

Michelle did well for a while, but as she continued to grow and eventually reached puberty, her anxiety again got the best of her. Coping skills were no longer enough and the lessons she had learned at age eight did not work for a teenager. Her mother made another appointment for Michelle, but this time with the pediatrician. This provider started her on a low dose anti-anxiety medication. In addition, she restarted counseling with a therapist more equipped to talk to adolescents.

Michelle's mother wondered if her daughter's anxiety was likely to be a lifelong ordeal. Would she need to remain on medication management? Would the medication change Michelle's personality? Would it cause long term side effects that affected her in adulthood? Would she require regular check-ins with a therapist?

Jennifer's Story

Jennifer started to prepare for her first year of high school. She loved reading and art. She was amazingly creative. The walls of her bedroom were lined with paintings she had crafted over several years. Jennifer was an introvert. She had a close friend she was bonded to, and they had survived elementary and middle school together. As summer was ending, Jennifer was excited by the promise of independence she believed came with being a high schooler. She became very disheartened when just before school was to begin, she learned her beloved friend was moving away.

Jennifer tried to remain optimistic. Her town had two middle schools, but only one high school. This meant she would likely meet a whole new group of teenagers she had never come into contact with before. Jennifer was hopeful she would find a new close friend. The first day of school she boarded the bus with a smile on her face.

High school was tougher than Jennifer thought it would be. Not only were the classes more challenging, but the social structure was foreign to her. She felt lonely sitting at lunch tables by herself and was scared to ask other classmates to team up with her for group projects. Finally, after three weeks of navigating the halls as a loner, she bumped into someone she had met previously in gymnastics.

Kelly was a beautiful girl. She had long, auburn wavy hair and appeared to have successfully navigated puberty without a hitch. This was very different than Jennifer who still wore braces, struggled with recurrent acne and had been given her mother's hair for which she described it as "frizzy and complicated." Jennifer wore glasses while Kelly's parents had agreed to get her contacts. Jennifer wore comfy clothes she had enjoyed picking out at a secondhand store and giving herself a personal style. Kelly bought new clothes from Abercrombie and Fitch or Forever 21 and seemed only to dress in the current season's line up. The girls didn't seem to care about their differences. They remembered the things they had in common in grade school and were able to rekindle their friendship.

Things had taken a turn for the better, Jennifer believed. She finally had connected with someone in high school. She no longer had to walk between classes alone or sit at a table for one during lunch. Everything was going great until Kelly announced she had a new boyfriend, Justin.

Justin was not the most popular guy in the ninth grade, but he did have a small group of friends. Many of these students were a grade ahead of him. Justin was happy avoiding homework and maintaining a C average. Kelly didn't care. She was infatuated by Justin, or at least the idea of having a high school boyfriend. Kelly began to spend more time with Justin and less time with Jennifer. This made Jennifer sad. She had enjoyed spending time with Kelly. Because of their close relationship she hadn't felt the need to socialize outside of their friendship.

Justin didn't mind if Jennifer hung out with him and Kelly. In fact, Kelly had started to get to know Justin's friends and the group would get together frequently in the evenings and weekends. One of the locations the teens frequented was the local park. This was great for Jennifer because she was within walking distance of the location. The teens met under a bridge for which they enjoyed spray painting the walls with colorful graffiti. At first, this made Jennifer uneasy. She had never done anything that was considered to be "wrong," but she wanted to be liked by her peers. The graffiti was not a bad thing she eventually determined. Who was going to see it? The location was remote. It was a slight hike to get back to their hangout from the main trail. Jennifer found it therapeutic to use the spray paint to create her own masterpiece on the brick wall.

As the group got to know Jennifer and Kelly better, they started to include them in other hobbies. While some of the activities were innocent, such as skateboarding, other activities were not as harmless. Under the influence of her new friends, Jennifer had stolen public property, tried marijuana, skipped school, and snuck a boy into her home for sexual activity, all within a few short months. Jennifer's parents were dismayed. The sweet girl they once knew had started acting out in ways they had not expected. Jennifer was defiant. She stopped turning in her homework. She started choosing inappropriate clothing selections to get attention from boys.

Jennifer started first with counseling. The weekly sessions didn't seem to be very effective. Due to the severity of the condition, her parents sought out medication management through a psychiatrist. Jennifer's aunt had a strong history of bipolar disorder and there was concern Jennifer was following in her footsteps. Jennifer was scheduled for specialist consultation early on in hopes that prompt addition of medication would help deter any future mental health ailments. The medication did not prove to be successful. Soon Jennifer started spending time in her bed and not wanting to leave her room. She would sleep the greater part of 16 hours. She did not talk with her family. Her hygiene became very poor, and she refused to shower. She stopped eating. The only thing that made Jennifer feel alive was time with her friends.

One night Jennifer decided to sneak out of the home and meet up with her friends. A new girl to the group, Kristen, drove up to Jennifer's house at midnight and Jennifer crawled out of a first-floor window to meet up with her. Kristen was 15, not old enough to have a driver's license. She had driven her mother's car to pick up Jennifer. Kristen's mother was unaware of the missing vehicle. Jennifer and Kristen picked up a few others and the friends partied into the night howling and laughing as the car flew down country roads. They celebrated their freedom with alcohol. The party ended when Kristen flipped the vehicle going too fast down a winding road. Thankfully, Jennifer left the scene with only a few bruises. When Jennifer's parents discovered what had happened, they were beside themselves. They knew Jennifer needed greater help to get her life turned around, but where would they start?

Josh's Story

"Do you want to come play a board game?" his mother asked.

"No," Josh mumbled in response.

Josh's room was dark. The window was covered by thick curtains. Only a small streak of light crept between the window coverings to illuminate the lump of adolescent body lying still in his bed. He was covered by a puffy blanket and faced his wall, his back to his mother.

"Have you showered today?" she questioned, already knowing the answer she would receive.

"I don't remember," Josh followed up.

The room was a disorganized mess. Clothes scattered the floor and piles of half completed projects lined his desk and dresser. There was a half-eaten plate of food sitting on his nightstand. Empty snack wrappers were strewn on the floor next to his bed. His mother moved from the hallway where she had been standing and into Josh's bedroom. "Time to get moving and be productive!" she exclaimed, throwing open the curtains. "You're not going to spend your Saturday just lying in bed. It's not good for you."

"I'm not getting out of bed," Josh grumbled. He grabbed the blanket from around his shoulders and covered his head trying to block out the light from the window.

"Not an option," his mother replied.

"Yes, it is. What are you going to do? I don't care if you take away my stuff. You cannot force me to do anything. Just ground me to my room and go away."

Josh's mother felt helpless. She knew her son struggled from depression. Josh's mood had worsened over the past few months. There wasn't a specific trigger that she was aware of that started the decline. Josh no longer was motivated to do things he used to enjoy, like walking the dog or seeing his friends. He occasionally left his room to get a snack but would return shortly after. He refused to go to therapy appointments she made for him. Josh was in middle school. If this is what the early teenage years looked like, what kind of future lay ahead for him?

Welcome to My Story

Mental wellness was not something that was regularly talked about in my household growing up. My father was a minister and both of my parents taught in the public school system. Their full-time job was reaching out to individuals in need and providing them with encouragement mentally, spiritually, and educationally. When it came to my own struggles with anxiety, depression, and an eating disorder I didn't feel I received the same support. I felt their attitude was, "These things don't happen to members of our family, only to others."

I remember trying to fall asleep in my canopy bed during my early years of elementary school. I could feel my heart racing as I thought through the events of the next day. I cried when I received a low grade on an assignment from my sixth-grade teacher. I tied my self-worth into perfectionism. I struggled maintaining close friendships from elementary through high school. I believed it was easier to change friend groups than to become vulnerable to anyone specific. I recall withholding food to lose weight and fit in during middle school. I lacked the knowledge of the effects of poor nutrition on a growing adolescent body. My elimination of food eventually caused fatigue, hair loss, and a lack nutrients to my body, leading to a condition known as anemia. By my junior year I had not only suicidal thoughts, but a well-developed scheme to escape my life. I'm not sure why I never acted on this plan. My parents did not recognize my battles with mental health. I was not offered counseling as a resource, let alone medication management.

I relied on hard work to get me through my studies. I feared failure above all other things. My anxiety drove my motivation to accomplish great tasks, but often got in my way and reduced my productivity. Frequently after finishing a task, my adrenaline would start to calm, and I would find myself in a world of depression. I didn't want to get out of bed, let alone engage with others. It was at the encouragement of a friend I first sought counseling services during my undergraduate years.

Over the past two decades I have learned just how much heredity and environmental components play in mental health. On some level, I will always need to be aware of my genetic predisposition. To be fully well I need to take active steps daily to work on boosting the chemicals in my brain that promote calmness. I also require a therapeutic technique known as mindfulness to help reduce stress that presents itself to me throughout the day. Growing up I felt my anxiety and depression were a handicap. Now I understand this past has given me an advantage. For years I have encountered many individuals with mental health ailments both professionally and in my own home. I feel my personal background and my training as a physician has allowed me to be more empathetic and skilled at providing care to these people.

Children come into our lives in many ways. There may be some individuals who start dreaming about raising a family when they are young. They enjoy interacting with children. They read books and study the "perfect parenting strategies." Other individuals may have stumbled into parenthood. They may not have planned on becoming a parent and found themselves one morning getting the news that in nine short months they would be responsible for another human being. Both as a mother, and as a healthcare professional, I have met parents from all walks of life. Being a parent is a challenging task. Each child is different and there is not a "one size fits all" model when it comes to addressing your child's needs. The process of guiding a child from infancy to young adulthood becomes even more difficult when you discover your child suffers from a mental health diagnosis.

I am a mother of a blended family. My husband brought two children to our relationship, and I brought three. There are three years and four months between the oldest of the clan and the youngest. We have two girls and three boys. All five children have struggled with a form of mental health wellness. For years I have relied heavily on learning from the knowledge of others. It was disheartening when I found little material written by parents on how best to handle the challenges of an adolescent struggling with mental health. In addition, the world of mental health resources is vast in variety and extremely small in availability. I felt lost. My desire is to have my children flourish as adults, but I had no idea where to begin. I have found treating a child with anxiety and depression is much different than seeking help personally or for an adult with the same diagnoses.

As a Family Medicine physician, I consider myself the "Marine of the Medicine World." The United States Marine Corps is recognized as one of the most elite forces in the world. The Marines are responsible for providing an ever-ready force to protect the U.S. interests anywhere in the world. The Marines typically lead the charge in military missions. Likewise, Family Medicine physicians are responsible for leading the care of their patients. As the Marines work on land, in the air, and in the water, Family Medicine physicians work on the physical, mental, and spiritual health of their patients.

Family Medicine can be rewarding because I get to lead the charge for adolescents' health. I have an opportunity to watch infants grow into adolescents and adults. Some of my patients have gone on to have children of their own and I'm blessed to care for their offspring. I work with the patients I serve to understand their social environment and provide resources for wellbeing based on the circumstance they find themselves in. I decipher whether an ailment is physical or emotional. I determine if specialty care is needed, or if I can take care of the patient's concerns based on my years of training. I have come to understand that with many of my patient's physical illnesses, there is an underlying mental health concern. While this is not always the case, it certainly is the situation more often than not.

I am a graduate of Michigan State University College of Osteopathic Medicine. I did my undergraduate studies in Physiology and Psychology, focusing heavily on brain development during adolescence. My residency after medical school was in Family Medicine. Currently in my outpatient clinic I treat infants through elderly patients. Many of the individuals I serve struggle with one or more mental health diagnoses. I am excited to share with you the knowledge I have gained while working with these patients as well as my own experience traversing the field of psychology to help myself and my family. To those parents who feel overwhelmed and defeated working with their children on a mental health journey, you are not alone.

Homework: Write your own family's experience. (Additional Matter – Your Story. Note: Google defines the "Appendix" as "the section of additional matter at the end of a book." I find the word "Appendix" to be boring and sadly, often skip over it when reading a text. Since I would like to invite you to complete the helpful assignments and absorb the content of the material from each chapter, from here on I will refer to the "Appendix" as "Additional Matter." It sounds so much more friendly, doesn't it?)

Chapter 2

NATURE VS. NURTURE

Which came first? The chicken? Or the egg? Evolutionary speaking, eggs existed before chickens (Fabry, 2016). Over 190 million years ago a creature with more than one cell began to develop specialized cells (Fabry, 2016). The exceptional cells could combine with the cells from another creature. Together, a new creature may be born. In other words, scientifically at some point in history there were no chickens. Two birds, that were almost, but not quite, chickens mated and laid an egg that hatched into the first chicken. If you think of that first egg as a chicken's egg, then the egg came before the chicken. On the other hand, a literal interpretation of the Bible would put the chicken before the egg. To quote the book of Genesis: "God blessed them and said to them, be fruitful and increase in number; fill the earth and subdue it. Rule over the fish in the sea and the birds in the sky and over every living creature that moves on the ground." (New International Version, Genesis 1:28). Aristotle supported the idea of the chicken being established before the egg. Aristotle deduced that actuality always comes before potentiality (Scott, 2003). So, the (actual) chicken came before the (potential) egg. Whether you believe the chicken came first, or you believe the egg came first, there is one thing I am certain. Both chickens and eggs are delicious. (Unless of course, as my son pointed out, you are vegan.)

As complicated as the debate about chickens and eggs may seem, the idea of your child's mental health coming from nature (their genetics), or nurture (their environment) is even more complex. Individuals do not fit a "one size fits all" mold. Every single human being is unique. Before we jump into the fascinating subject of how physical, environmental, and spiritual health can influence our mental wellbeing, let's go over a few key concepts of human biology. (Don't worry, there isn't a test at the end of the chapter!)

The Basics of Genetics

Genes are the blueprints of cells within the body (Greenblatt & Lee, 2019). Genes tell a cell how to form and how to function. You inherited one set of genes from your mother and another set of genes from your father and they combined to create a lovely being… you! Each gene is made of two polynucleotide chains coiled around one another to form a double helix known as deoxyribonucleic acid (DNA). There are approximately 20,000 to 25,000 genes in the human genome (the name for the entire gene collection of an individual) (MedlinePlus, 2021). Genes may vary in size. Not all genes are active at any given time (Greenblatt & Lee, 2019). When the body needs a specific gene, the gene turns on and "uncoils" the necessary DNA so it can be acted upon. After the gene has completed its needed function, the gene turns off and recoils itself to remain hidden again until it is needed in the future. An individual may inherit a gene from a parent that presents as depression or anxiety, however, the gene is not necessarily turned "on" (Greenblatt & Ross-Taylor, 2019).

In determining the extent that genetics plays a role in mental health, researchers have frequently studied identical twins. Identical twins come from a single egg that has been fertilized and splits in two. The twins have the same DNA. Scientists will look for an individual who suffers from mental health and has an identical twin. The mental wellbeing of the twins will be compared. The identical twins have the same genetic material but have been exposed to different environmental factors, since no two individuals experience the world in the same way. In many cases, after reviewing the data, genetic influence was found to be a predictor of long-term mental health (Greenblatt & Ross-Taylor, 2019).

Perhaps genes should be thought of as "recommendations." The genetic code is present, but how an individual chooses to immerse themselves in their environment decides whether the gene turns on fully, partially, or not at all. According to genetic theory, genes are stable (Agutter, 2007). Significant changes to the genetic code are only likely to occur as a means of species survival. Alterations to genes take place at a very slow rate. It may take hundreds or even millions of years before inherited mutations are observed (Agutter, 2007). If an individual develops a medical illness during their lifetime, such as diabetes, this single event will not drastically change the genetic map of future offspring. If, however, generations of individuals all became diabetic because of the food sources available, their DNA may evolve to better metabolize the nutrients at hand.

Epigenetics is a term used to describe the study of how your behaviors and environment can lead to changes that affect the way your genes work (Greenblatt & Ross-Taylor, 2019). When an individual is affected by an external stressor, whether that be related to a disease, a change in nutrition, physical or emotional stress, drugs, or any other outside factor, a gene may be turned on or turned off (Greenblatt & Lee, 2019). Outside stimuli can therefore be responsible for genetic code expression.

To better understand epigenetics, let's picture a traffic signal. A traffic light consists of a red light, a yellow light, and a green light. In their simplest form, traffic signals face each lane of an intersection. When the light is green, that lane has the right of way to cross. When the light is red, the lane may not cross. When the light is yellow, it tells drivers to watch out, the light is about to turn red. To help facilitate traffic at a junction of road, when your light is red, the intersecting traffic's light is green so that they can cross safely. Your light will turn green when it is safe for you to travel.

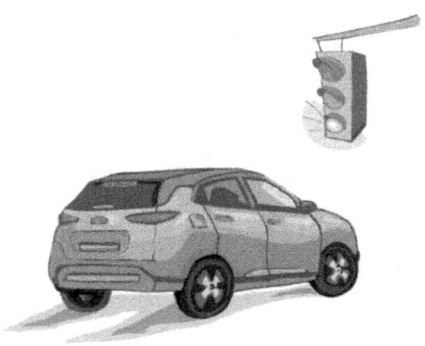

Now, for this example, let's say the traffic lights are on a timer. The timer tells the traffic signal when to change color, like the body tells the genetic code when to turn on or turn off. When the timer works, the flow of traffic is seamless. But what if the timer were to stop working? Your traffic light rotates between green, yellow, and red lights on a whim. The same thing occurs with the crossing traffic's signal. There is no correlation between your light and the crossing traffic light. Suddenly your light is green, and the crossing traffic light is green. Both cars at the intersection take off. Crash! Epigenetics, like the non-working timer, took the lead and became the narrator of telling the genetic code (traffic light) when to turn "on" and "off." The body was not in charge of the genetic code and the result was a nasty fender bender between two cars.

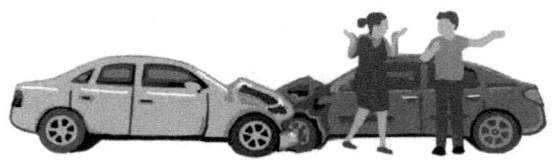

So back to our original question. What is responsible for your child's mental health? You? Or the environment? The answer is yes. Both genetics and the environment play a supporting role in your child's development (Greenblatt & Ross-Taylor, 2019). You provided a genetic code, as did your partner, and the two codes were woven into a precious zygote (a single celled organism resulting from a fertilized egg) which rapidly became a developing embryo (the early stage of human development where critical body organs are formed). At approximately six to ten days after fertilization, the embryo implants itself into the uterine lining. The embryo begins receiving its nourishment and oxygen from the cells along the uterine wall. If a woman's uterine lining has been affected by her hormones or medications she is ingesting, the lining may not be thick enough for the embryo to attach itself to. Even in this primal state, epigenetics is already starting to affect the growing child.

The brain begins to develop during the third week of gestation, also known as the seventh week of pregnancy (What to Expect, 2021). Neural progenitor cells begin to divide and differentiate into neurons and glia, the two cell types that form the basis of the nervous system. By the ninth week, the brain appears as a small, smooth structure (What to Expect, 2021). In my experience, most women discover they are pregnant between weeks four and seven of pregnancy.

If a woman smokes or drinks alcohol, she may not have sufficient oxygen levels or vitamins to feed the growing baby's brain (Farber & Olney, 2003). When neuronal activity is abnormally suppressed during the developmental period, the timing and sequence of chemical and electrical connections between brain cells is disrupted. This disruption may cause nerve cells to receive an internal signal to commit suicide, a form of cell death known as apoptosis. Alcohol, for instance, alters glutamate and gamma aminobutyric acid (GABA) transmission (Farber & Olney, 2003). These substances are naturally occurring amino acids that work as neurotransmitters (chemical messengers) in your brain. When glutamate and GABA transmission has been changed, they signal to increase cell death. This proapoptotic effect of alcohol, and many other drugs of abuse, during brain development may explain the decreased brain size and lifelong neurobehavioral disturbances associated with conditions such as fetal alcohol syndrome (Farber & Olney, 2003).

Emotional responses triggered by abuse, anxiety, depression, lack of sleep, and reduced appetite can have health risks for a pregnant woman and her developing baby. The American College of Obstetricians and Gynecologists (ACOG) reports that one in six abused women are first abused during pregnancy. More than 320,000 women are abused by their partners during pregnancy each year (ACOG, 2012). A population-based study published in *JAMA Psychiatry* reported that children of women who experience depression during pregnancy are 1.5 times more likely to be depressed themselves as teenagers (Krans, 2013).

Once an infant emerges into the world, the quality of their postnatal environment is shaped by interactions, especially parent-offspring contact, that may lead to divergent developmental trajectories with implications for later-life neurobiological and behavioral characteristics. New technology in the fields of molecular biology and brain imaging have helped point towards pathways (such as exposure to toxins, nutritional variation, and stress) which may be similar in early-life experiences. Knowing how these events can alter a child's brain development allows researchers to begin to identify the mechanism underlying the impact of parents on their children. In a review published in *Neuropsychopharmacology*, Drs. Kundakovic and Champagne note, "In particular, it is evident that the quality of parent-offspring interaction induces epigenetic changes in the developing brain that account for variation in response to stress, cognition, sociality, and reproductive behavior" (Kundakovic & Champagne, 2015).

Technology and Mental Health

There is a growing mountain of evidence showing significant clinical and neurological consequences of digital technology on mental health (Kardaras, 2016). Generation Y, or Millennials, were the first generation to grow up with the internet, cell phones, and digital communication. Technology has brought some great advancements. For instance, the digital world allowed for more convenient communication, the healthcare industry to improve its efficiency, and enhanced learning opportunities by way of easier access. Advancements in technology have also come at a cost. Children who overuse technology may be more likely to experience low academic performance, language delay, poor sleep quality, inattention, anxiety, depression, and increased health risks, such as obesity and vision impairment (Regis College, 2021). A research article published in JAMA Pediatrics noted that prior to the 2020 coronavirus pandemic, United States adolescents ages 10 to 14 reported almost four hours a day of technology time (Nagata, et. al, 2022). That number increased to nearly eight hours a day in the same individuals during the pandemic. Despite the gradual reversal of quarantine restrictions, technology use has remained elevated (Nagata, et. al, 2022). In addition, children have spent more time isolated from their peers. Include the racial tensions, divisive political upheaval and other social issues posted online in the past two years, it is of no surprise that the number of adolescents reporting irritability, anxiety, and depression has gone up dramatically.

Dr. Kardaras explored the world of technology in his book, *Glow Kids*. He reports, "Perhaps most shocking of all, recent brain-imaging studies conclusively show that excessive screen exposure can neurologically damage a young person's developing brain in the same way that cocaine addiction can. That's right – a kid's brain on tech looks like a brain on drugs" (Kardaras, 2016). For decades schools have declared a so-called "War on Drugs," yet we've allowed what Chinese researchers call "electronic heroine" to slip into our homes and schools (Kardaras, 2016). Technology is affecting our youngest and most vulnerable. Many well-meaning parents are oblivious to the ill effects of increased screen time. Sadly, while some parents do recognize the damaging effects digital time may have, they remain in convenience-induced denial (Kardaras, 2016).

I believe social media and video games contribute to the increasing mental illness in the United States. Dopamine, a chemical messenger in the brain, is released when the brain is expecting, or receives, a reward. When you come to associate a certain activity with pleasure, mere anticipation may be enough to raise dopamine levels. Think about the "like" status on social media. Let's say an adolescent girl posts a selfie on Instagram. Her friends "like" her status. Soon she has 153 "likes." Her dopamine begins to climb as she feels positive feedback on her post from her peers. Three hours later, however, she no longer feels the pleasure from her Instagram status as her dopamine levels reduce. The girl feels the need to post another picture. Dopamine again increases making her feel happiness as she awaits the rising number of "likes" from her peers. This time she received 86 "likes." This number was lower. "What did I do wrong?" she thinks. She tries to be more extreme with her next post and only waits an hour before posting it to try and feel better.

Individuals may receive a similar dopamine rush when they experience hyperarousal while playing video games. The brain links increased levels of dopamine during the activity to a feeling of enjoyment. When the individual's dopamine begins to wane, it's likely they will have a strong drive to seek out video games again and again.

Unfortunately, in both the scenario with social media, and the situation with video games, as the outside influence takes over the dopamine response within the body, epigenetics downregulates the body's ability to make and release its own dopamine. The production of dopamine may reduce or the sensors for dopamine uptake may become less sensitive. Subsequently, the individual needs to return to the activity to make up for the pleasure the body can no longer derive on its own (Greenblatt & Ross-Taylor, 2019). I've frequently tried to relay the biochemical consequences to my patients. Often, parents are grateful their child is safe in their room "communicating with others" or "playing games" and not out on the streets seeking drugs and alcohol. But is this really a safe option?

Nutrition and Mental Health

In my training as an osteopathic physician, a great emphasis was placed on the connection between mind and body. Over the past decade, I have come to appreciate the strong connection between mental wellbeing and nutrition. In an adult, the average brain utilizes 20% of the body's energy (Greenblatt & Lee, 2019). This means that different mental states and tasks can subtly affect the way the brain consumes energy. In a child, the brain is rapidly developing. During some growth states, the brain may utilize as much as 50% of the body's energy (ScienceDaily, 2019). It goes back to the nineteenth century saying, "You are what you eat."

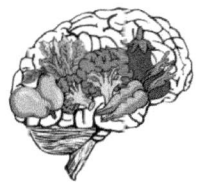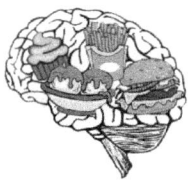

In the past decade, bestselling books like *Grain Brain* and *Wheat Belly*, that describe elimination of gluten and dietary trends, like veganism, that eliminate dairy, have become popular in mental health. Can foods that have been an essential and nourishing part of the human diet for thousands of years really be that bad for mental health? My answer is, in some individuals they can.

Grains like wheat, oats, rye, and barley contain a protein called gluten. In the body gluten becomes gliadorphin (Greenblatt & Gottlieb, 2017).

Dairy foods like milk, cheese, and butter contain a protein called casein. In the body casein becomes casomorphin (Greenblatt & Gottlieb, 2017).

Why is this important? Gliadorphin and casomorphin attach to opiate receptors in the brain. Opiate receptors are part of the endogenous opioid system, which is the body's internal system for regulating pain, reward, and addictive behaviors (Greenblatt & Gottlieb, 2017). If you are wondering, "Are these the same opiate receptors I've heard about with substances like morphine?" You are correct! As their names indicate, both gliadorphin and casomorphin are morphinelike compounds. Many parents would not willingly give their adolescent pain medication, such as morphine, several times a day. The long-term effects would include brain fog, fatigue, irritability and aggression, anxiety, depression, and insomnia! Yet many of us start our children's day before school with a bowl of tasty Cinnamon Toast Crunch drenched in delicious cow's milk. Now, that does not mean that we are poisoning every child who enjoys cereal in the morning. As I mentioned previously, every individual is unique. While the epigenomes of several children may not be "turned on" by gluten or dairy, in my experience, there are a great number of children who are affected.

Sleep and Mental Health

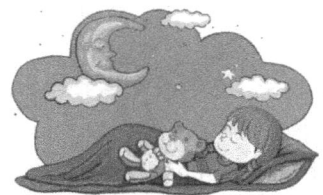

The brain and the body need sleep to fully recharge and restore maximum functioning. A lack of sleep can affect the brain by leading to increased irritability, slower thinking, and depression (Greenblatt & Lee, 2019). It can also cause increased blood pressure, diabetes, heart disease, obesity, and reduced immunity within the body. Problems with sleep may be caused by poor sleep hygiene, nutritional imbalances, and physical ailments (Greenblatt & Lee, 2019). Sleep is especially critical for the adolescent population. Children between five and twelve years of age need about ten to eleven hours of sleep each night. When the brain does not get time to rest it can cause neurotransmitter and hormone changes that affect the neuronal network (Greenblatt & Lee, 2019). In my medical practice, children with sleep problems often have a higher prevalence of generalized anxiety disorder, depression, inattention, and other behavioral conditions.

Chronic Illness and Mental Health

Physical ailments can influence mood. In a 2015 Canadian study, inflammatory response in the areas of the brain dealing with emotional regulation were 30% higher in those who were clinically depressed (Greenblatt & Lee, 2019). When an individual faces a significant injury or infection, the body produces chemicals called pro-inflammatory cytokines. The increased release of cytokines signals the immune system to wake up and begin its job of restoring balance in the body. Unfortunately, cytokines may also stimulate the release of certain neurotransmitters. When the body sees increased neurotransmitters in the brain, it reduces production of those substances. When the supply of neurotransmitters is less than the demand for neurotransmitters, depression or other mental illnesses may result (Greenblatt & Lee, 2019).

Spirituality and Mental Health

The idea of spirituality means different things for different people, but across the board, spirituality has a profound effect on mental health. Spirituality is not the same as religion. Spirituality is a connectedness within oneself, between yourself and others, between yourself and your environment, and between yourself and the unknown. Religion is a particular system of faith and worship. Spirituality can help you deal with stress by giving you a sense of purpose and a feeling of peace. When I talk to patients who are struggling with mental health, they often feel disconnected from others and isolated. They report feelings of chaos from within. One way individuals may connect to spiritually is through meditation. A 2017 Harvard Medical School study showed that after meditating 15 minutes daily for eight weeks, the meditators had changes in 172 genes that control inflammation, sleep-wake rhythms in the body and how the body processes sugar (Health and Wellness, 2018).

The study of epigenetics creates a matrix of the previous nature versus nurture debate. Epigenetic changes based on one's environmental experience allows everyone to be biochemically unique (Greenblatt & Lee, 2019). This means no two cases of mental illness can be exactly the same. Currently, scientists have not been able to pinpoint a specific epigenomic modification to a resulting mental health ailment. As such, there is no one medication, diet, or therapy that is universal. Mental health treatment is uniquely tailored to an individual. My hope is knowing this fact will bring you comfort and hope as you support your child on their wellness journey.

Chapter 2 Summary

- Individuals do not fit a "one size fits all" mold.

- Physical, environmental, and spiritual health can influence our mental wellbeing.

- Genes are the blueprints of cells within the body. Not all genes are active at any given time. An individual may inherit a gene from a parent that presents as a mental ailment, however, the gene is not necessarily turned "on."

- No two individuals experience the world in the same way. Epigenetics is a term used to describe the study of how your behaviors and environment can lead to changes that affect the way your genes work.

- Epigenetics begins to affect the growing child even during early pregnancy.

- There is growing evidence showing significant clinical and neurological consequences of digital technology on mental health.

- What an individual eats, how much sleep an individual receives on a regular basis, and an individual's chronic health issues may affect mental health.

- Spirituality can help an individual manage daily stress by giving them a feeling of connectedness.

Homework: Identify internal and external factors affecting your family. (Additional Matter – Factors Affecting Your Family's Mental Health)

Chapter 3

THE HEDGE MAZE OF THE BEHAVIORAL HEALTH SYSTEM

I recall my first time walking through the "baby section" of the grocery store. So many items for such a small person. It was a little intimidating. Formulas, first step foods, diapers, wipes, pacifiers, and bottles. Where would I even begin? Was there that much of a difference between Enfamil, Similac and Gerber? Would my child be ruined forever if I bought them a pacifier? Was I to purchase glass bottles, plastic bottles, or bottles with liners? If I did choose the right bottle, would it go with "slow bottle nipples" or "fast bottle nipples"? Was there a difference between applesauce in the main grocery aisle and applesauce in the baby aisle besides the price? I suspect you had a similar experience the first time you brought your bundle of joy into the world. Even if it wasn't the supermarket, maybe it was determining the right car seat, stroller, crib, play pen, or highchair. Whether in the end you chose Pampers, Huggies, Luvs, or cloth diapers, you and your child eventually made it through those early years.

Since there is no aisle of behavioral health services at the local store, initially the behavioral health system does not seem so daunting. From my medical school training I knew the difference between a psychologist (a doctor with a PhD or PsyD who is an expert on the mind and behavior) and a psychiatrist (a medical doctor with a MD or DO who treats mental health, most often, with medication). I also knew the difference between outpatient services (non-hospital based) and inpatient services (hospital based). I was taught some basic psychological diagnoses and medications, but at most, it was a mere introduction to this very important world of mental wellbeing.

I titled this chapter "The Hedge Maze of the Behavioral Health System." For those who may be unfamiliar, a hedge maze is an outdoor garden maze, or labyrinth, in which the "walls" or dividers between passages are made of vertical hedges. A hedge maze is complex and often individuals find themselves confused when traveling from point A to point B. Individuals suffering from mental health ailments are vulnerable and often struggling with regular activities of daily living. Yet, the behavioral health system in many cases is one of the most complex systems to find the right services.

Some children are just easier to raise than others. Tim Thayne, a psychologist who has devoted his life to helping struggling adolescents, explains this well in his book, *Not by Chance*. According to Dr. Thayne, raising easy children is like hitting a five-foot bullseye from 20 feet away (Thayne, 2013). When it comes to these adolescents, many parents can be loving, involved, and consistent and those children will "turn out" just fine. Fortunately, these teens will keep most of the rules most of the time. They'll accept "no" without too much push back. They'll do well in school and require moderate encouragement to keep them moving in the right direction. Overall, basic parenting will be sufficient for these children (Thayne, 2013).

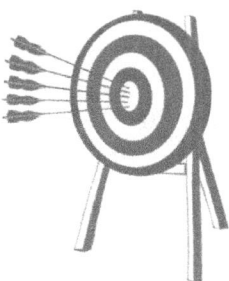

Not all children are quite so easy. Some have challenging temperaments. Others may battle with mental health. Dr. Thayne notes that parenting these children is like hitting a one-foot bullseye from 20 feet away (Thayne, 2013). That does not mean that we accept difficult children are hard to raise and leave it at that. It means that as parents, we want to learn, practice, and refine our skills until we become good at hitting that one-foot bullseye. This may mean finding the right provider in your community for your struggling youth (Thayne, 2013). In extreme cases, it may mean finding a program 1300 miles away to help your child thrive. While the last one may seem a little excessive, it was the best thing we could have done for one of my children.

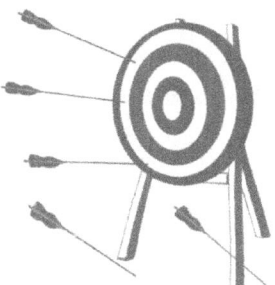

If you're reading this book, most likely you have already stepped foot into the pool of behavioral services. Perhaps you are in the shallow end of the pool, not realizing the depth of treatments available, but knowing what you've encountered this far is not working for your family. It's possible you jumped into the deep end of the pool and are aware of the number of treatments out there, but unsure how to swim to the one that fits your needs. In this chapter I'm going to need you to take a step back from the pool. Find a cozy spot on a deck chair. Grab your favorite umbrella drink. Let's look at the pool from an aerial view.

Employee Assistance Program (EAP)

Definition: An employee benefit program that helps workers with personal problems that may impact their job performance, health, mental, and emotional well-being (SHRM 2022).

Two months ago, twelve-year-old Nichole started middle school. She had excelled in her elementary school classes, but transitioning to multiple teachers, harder material, and increasing homework was overwhelming for her. Nichole had not previously needed skills in organization and time management, but her new schedule required a fresh approach. Nichole's mother thought her daughter may benefit from short term counseling services, so she contacted her human resources department to see what benefits were available.

As a parent, you may work for a company that invests in an employee assistance program (EAP). An EAP is a voluntary, work-based program that offers free and confidential assessments, short-term counseling, referrals, and follow-up services (U.S. OPM, 2022). Employers pay a provider to offer resources to their workers. These resources do not get billed through employee insurance. The employer does not know who utilized resources, only those resources provided. The benefit to the employer is that employees who participate in EAP programs typically miss less time at work. The employees can get the help they need, often after hours. Regarding counseling services, I have seen as little as four sessions and as many as twelve sessions be available through EAPs. If a situation requires more than the allowable EAP benefit, the provider will often bridge the gap as additional services are arranged.

Who's Who of Behavioral Health

Primary Care Provider (PCP)

Definition: A primary care provider is a medical professional who may be both the first contact for an individual with an undiagnosed health concern, as well as providing continued care of varied medical conditions. For a child, this may be a pediatrician or a family medicine physician. In some cases, a PCP may be an advanced practice provider (APP). A primary care physician typically has completed eleven years of training or more beyond high school and has a degree as a MD (Doctor of Medicine) or DO (Doctor of Osteopathic Medicine). An advanced practice provider typically has completed six years of training or more beyond high school and has a degree as a NP (Nurse Practitioner) or PA (Physician Assistant).

Cost: According to a study by the Agency for Healthcare Research and Quality, the mean expense for primary care specialties without insurance coverage is $186, and the median expense is $107. If you are covered by insurance, the average cost that is paid out-of-pocket is significantly cheaper, with a mean of $50 and a median of $25. Many provider offices have payment plans available if requested (Fazio, 2021).

How to Find Services:

1. Your health insurance plan. Your health insurance plan may keep an online list of network primary care providers who are accepting new patients.

2. Personal referrals. People often ask their friends, families, and co-workers for referral to primary care physicians. If someone you respect and trust has a positive experience with a doctor, it's

possible you may like that physician. I often see requests for referrals on local social media sites in my area as well.

3. Referrals from your current physician. If you are moving to a new area, you could ask your current provider to help you find a primary care physician in your new neighborhood.

4. Hospital access. It is common for hospitals to offer a referral service that can provide the names of staff doctors who meet certain criteria you may be seeking, such as specialty, gender, experience, and location.

Rick is 14 years old. He has missed nearly two weeks of school this semester. When Rick is absent, it's generally because of headaches, stomach aches, or fatigue. He no longer finds interest in activities he used to enjoy. He would rather lay in bed than socialize with his friends. Rick has been eating less and not sleeping well at night. Rick's mother has a history of depression, and his father is concerned Rick may be experiencing similar behavioral patterns. His father schedules an appointment with the pediatrician to find out what to do next.

Over the past five years I have had more and more patients like Rick show up in my office. If identified early enough, many children respond well to counseling sessions and medication management is not needed. The number of sessions required by a child to obtain wellness varies. Some children require six weekly sessions and then check in with their provider as needed. Other children require bi-weekly sessions for a year or more. It's often of great benefit for adolescents to have an adult that is not a family member to discuss the challenges they face. Teens especially may be more open to communicate with a counselor than their own parents.

Behavioral Health Consultant (BHC)

Definition: A behavioral consultant works with patients to address and improve behavior concerns. A BHC assesses each patient's mental health and creates a treatment plan to reduce negative behavior and promote positive choices.

Cost: The average cost of therapy is $60 to $150 per session, with most American's paying between $20 and $250 per hour depending on the number of sessions booked, and if it's covered by health insurance. With health insurance coverage, rates average $20 to $50 per session, or about equal to your current copay (BikeHike, 2022).

How to Find Services: Most commonly, referrals will come from your PCP, however, additional ways to find a counselor include: through your insurance provider, asking friends, family and co-workers, and hospital access.

I am blessed to have a behavioral health consultant (BHC) in my medical practice. My BHC can provide several services to my patients. For instance, I have referred patients to my BHC for counseling on smoking cessation, understanding triggers to unhealthy habits, and bereavement. I have had my BHC assess patients' mental health to provide a more in-depth evaluation on anxiety, depression, inattention, and trauma. My BHC has provided short-term therapy to teach mindfulness and emotional regulation skills. When psychotherapy does not seem to be enough, I work with my BHC to get a better understanding of the patient and am more equipped to prescribe the appropriate medication. My BHC helps follow patients in crises. When additional resources are needed, my BHC helps bridge the gap to longer term therapeutic providers. In healthcare, BHCs often are licensed clinical social workers.

Licensed Clinical Social Worker (LCSW)

Definition: An individual who has completed at least two years of clinically supervised full-time postgraduate experience providing direct clinical support. They may assess, diagnose, and provide treatment for emotional and behavioral concerns. They are expected to fulfill requirements in their state of practice to obtain licensure and must also successfully pass a national examination. Some states call these individuals LICSWs (licensed independent clinical social workers) (Ardito, 2020).

Cost: LCSWs can practice independently and receive reimbursement from insurance companies for psychotherapy and counseling services. Not all LCSWs accept insurance, and some require a fee-for-service where direct payment is expected from the client. A typical therapy session with a LCSW can cost $80 to $150 per hour (Ardito, 2020).

How to Find Services: If you are planning to use insurance benefits for psychotherapy, it may be helpful to contact your insurance company directly about in-network providers. Many insurance companies now offer an online resource to search for services within a particular geographical location. Your PCP may have counselors they frequently refer to. Psychology Today is a well-known database for finding therapists as well.

Other Types of Therapist Credentials

LCAT: Licensed Creative Arts Therapist

LMFT: Licensed Marriage and Family Therapist

LMHC: Licensed Mental Health Counselor

LMSW: Licensed Master Social Work

PhD or PsyD, HSSP: Clinical Psychologist with an endorsement as a Health Service Provider in Psychology

Your chosen therapist may have different credentials but must be licensed to provide mental health treatment to be lawfully and ethically practicing providers. Your therapist will verify they are actively licensed by showing the "L" with their credential. They may even display their license at their work site.

For progress to be made, a counselor and their patient must have a good therapeutic relationship. Not every provider/client pair is a good fit. Personally, it wasn't until my fourth LCSW that I was able to successfully explore my own mental health battles and find peace. As a rule, I recommend three to four sessions with a therapist before determining if the "fit" is appropriate.

Remember Rick? After meeting with the pediatrician, the physician referred Rick to the BHC within the office. The BHC reached out by phone to Rick's father the next day and recommended several counselors that took Rick's insurance and were available after Rick got out of school. The BHC followed up with Rick's father two weeks later to be sure an appointment had been made, and even called after the first counseling appointment to be sure there were no new issues that came up in the interim and the first experience had gone well.

Rick met with the LCSW weekly for several weeks. After six weeks of treatment, Rick had made little improvement in what seemed like depression. The LCSW communicated with the pediatrician their concerns and recommended medication management. The pediatrician scheduled an appointment with Rick and his father and discussed the pros and cons of medication. The pediatrician recommended a group of medications called selective serotonin reuptake inhibitors (SSRIs). Rick was started on a low dose medication for his mood and a follow up appointment with the doctor was made for three weeks later.

At first Rick showed no changes in his behavior. Like the therapy he continued to participate in, the medication had little effect. About week two Rick started showing signs of overactivity and euphoria. Rick also started engaging with a concerning peer group at school. Rick's father contacted the pediatrician immediately. As this was generally not the response most patients had from this medication, it was recommended to discontinue the prescription immediately. The pediatrician reached out to an adolescent psychiatrist for evaluation and treatment.

Psychiatrist

Definition: A medical physician specializing in the diagnosis and treatment of mental illness. A psychiatrist can prescribe medication. They typically have twelve years of training or more after high school and are licensed as a MD or DO. An APP, such as an NP or PA, may also work in the psychiatry field.

Cost: According to Electronic Health Reporter, the average cost of a psychiatrist visit generally runs somewhere between $100 and $200 per session, but the initial appointment is often more. The first visit is often longer, and the specialist's workload is increased when seeing a patient for the first time. The doctor may need to order lab work or additional testing. Gathering and reviewing past documents regarding a patient's medical health is also necessary for proper treatment. Expect to pay about $300 - $500 for an initial consultation. Any specialized treatments, prescribed tests, bloodwork, and medications will be at an additional cost (Rice, 2021).

How to Find Services: Like PCPs and LCSWs, referrals generally come from other providers, acquaintances, and hospital access systems. You can also check your online insurance portal for in-network providers or check out the American Psychiatric Association's "Find a Psychiatrist" page (https://finder.psychiatry.org/).

The psychiatrist met with Rick and his father. He reviewed the notes from the pediatrician and counselor that had fortunately been forwarded ahead of Rick's initial appointment. The physician understood that counseling had not reached the desired response in elevating Rick's mood, and the usual prescribed medication caused significant side effects. The provider ordered laboratory testing to see there was an undiagnosed physiological cause. The blood work included: a complete blood count, thyroid studies, a complete metabolic panel, and vitamin studies. (Note, it is not uncommon for psychiatrists to investigate sleep habits by requesting a sleep study, food sensitivity testing to determine if there is a nutritional concern, or imaging scans to look at the anatomy of the brain.)

During the time that it took to receive the results of the additional testing, Rick started engaging in new behaviors. He was caught sneaking out of school to smoke marijuana under the sports bleachers on the football field. His parents were also called by the local police department when Rick was caught shoplifting at the mall. Grounding Rick to his room and separating him from spending time with his friends did not seem to motivate Rick to want to change his behavior. Rick did not appear to mind spending time alone and used the opportunity to sleep or put in his earbuds and listen to his music. When Rick and his father followed up with the psychiatrist, the provider reviewed Rick's symptoms. Rick's diagnosis was not clear cut. He exhibited features of several different mental health ailments. The psychiatrist ordered a full psychological examination with a local psychologist.

A Word About Insurance

If you have insurance, whether your provider is in- or out-of-network will have the largest impact on your overall treatment costs. In-network providers are generally much cheaper. Your insurer can provide you with a list of in-network providers, or you can contact a provider's office directly and see whether they accept your insurance provider. After these considerations, what you pay will ultimately be determined by how your out-of-pocket expenses are calculated.

Deductible: A deductible is how much you need to pay out of pocket before your insurance coverage kicks in. Until you reach the amount, you'll be covering the cost of your medical bills. A deductible may be a percentage, but most often it is a stated dollar amount. For example, if your deductible is $2500, you'll pay $2500 before your insurance starts to pay for any of your visits or treatments (Davalon, 2021).

Copay: A co-pay, short for co-payment, is a flat fee that you pay your provider for visits. This is a fixed amount determined by your insurance provider and it'll be the amount that you can expect to pay any visit. Co-pays may fluctuate depending on the type of insurance, type of provider, type of service, and type of appointment (Davalon, 2021). A primary care provider may have a co-pay of $20, whereas a psychiatrist may have a co-pay of $35.

Coinsurance: Coinsurance refers to the amount you pay for covered healthcare after you have paid your deductible (Davalon, 2021).

Psychologist

Definition: A doctor who studies cognitive, emotional, and social processes and behavior by observing, interpreting, and recording how people relate to one another and to their environments (Psychologists, 2022). A psychologist cannot prescribe medication. They typically have eight to twelve years of training after high school and have a Doctor of Philosophy (PhD), Doctor of Psychology (PsyD), or an education specialist degree (EdS).

Cost: On average, a visit with a psychologist, without health insurance, can cost anywhere from $75 to $200+ per hour (Devlin, 2022). As with a psychiatrist, the initial consultation with a psychologist may cost more. If a patient is receiving a psychological examination for the purposes of

> diagnosis and treatment plan, there may also be a flat rate for the service. I have seen psychological evaluations range between $1200 and $4000. Insurance may cover a portion of this testing.

Rick met with the psychologist on two separate occasions. Each session was approximately four hours. At the end of the testing, the psychologist provided Rick and his parents a full treatment plan that could be used by Rick's psychiatrist, pediatrician, counselor, and even school, to help Rick succeed. The treatment plan covered Rick's history, psychological testing/scores/and interpretation of results, diagnoses, and suggestions for behavioral services.

Where do Behavioral Health Services Take Place?

Behavioral health services may take place in a multitude of locations. The location of the service often depends on the type and intensity of treatment that is needed. Providers may meet with your child at home or at school. Counselors may have a specific office they work out of. Services that take place outside of a hospital system are known as "*outpatient services.*"

When a Child Needs Outpatient Services

Brandon is 15 years old. He sees his school counselor every Wednesday. He has been struggling with depression for some time. His doctor prescribed him Zoloft (sertraline) 200mg at night. He does not find enjoyment in seeing his friends. He cries in his room frequently. It's everything he can do just to get up and go to school each day. Brandon no longer turns in his homework. He frequently skips meals. His parents have tried to encourage him to do things with them, but Brandon declines. Brandon feels hopeless. He doesn't think anyone can help him. Nothing is working.

When weekly contact with a provider is not enough and an adolescent is in emotional crisis to the point it disrupts daily life at home or school, extra support can be provided through *intensive outpatient (IOP)* facilities. IOPs are treatment programs used to address addictions, depression, eating disorders, or other dependencies that do not require detoxification or round-the-clock supervision (American Addiction Center, 2022). Patients who attend IOPs live at home. Many IOP programs meet three hours at a time, three days a week. Patients participate in group therapy. They may also receive individual and family therapy. They can be evaluated by a psychiatrist for medication evaluation and treatment. IOPs can cost $250 to $350 per day depending on the program (Thomas, 2021). Individuals typically attend for eight to twelve weeks. Upon discharge from an IOP, individuals follow up with their previous healthcare team (counselor and doctor).

When a Child Needs More than Outpatient Services

Lizzy is 19 years old. She hasn't left her apartment in two weeks. She has been utilizing various illicit substances over the past three years, but most recently she started using heroin. She doesn't have any money. If Lizzy does happen to have an appetite, she struggles to find food. Her roommates come and go, but no one has noticed Lizzy's recent behaviors because she's been secluded to her room. Lizzy's boyfriend recently broke up with her which sent her into her last using spree. She's not shown up for her job. Her clothes are stained. She hasn't showered in days. She picks up her phone and calls her mom crying. "I don't want to live any more. I want to die!"

If an emotional crisis requires around-the-clock supervision, as is the case with detoxification, suicidal or homicidal thoughts and plan, a patient may be admitted to *"inpatient services."* Inpatient services take place within the hospital system. Individuals participate in regular individual, group, and family sessions. Psychiatrists make regular adjustments to medication. Individuals are kept in the hospital anywhere from a few days to a few weeks. Inpatient services help stabilize an individual from the emergent need. The length of time depends on the specific needs of the patient. Cost for inpatient services can be considerably variable depending on the reason the individual is admitted for treatment, the duration of treatment, and the services provided.

When the individual is ready to leave inpatient treatment, a "step-down" approach is typically appropriate. Patient's being discharged from inpatient, generally move down to *partial hospitalization programs (PHPs)*. While admitted to a PHP, the individual lives at home, but participates with behavioral health providers generally eight hours a day for five days a week, for two to four weeks, typically at a hospital setting. Once the healthcare team feels the patient is ready to move from PHP, they step-down to IOP, then back to their previous outpatient services.

Not all individuals are able to go from inpatient hospitalization to PHP. Sometimes a *residential* setting is more appropriate. A psychiatric residential treatment facility, or PRTF, is defined as a facility, other than a hospital, that provides live-in psychiatric services. For some adolescents, a *therapeutic boarding school* is an appropriate choice after inpatient stabilization. The therapy in a therapeutic boarding school is integrated into the classroom and all other daily activities. A team of teachers, therapists, and residential staff work together to help students achieve their treatment goals, while providing the structure necessary for success. These schools typically offer small classroom sizes, individualized plans, and academic support to help a student thrive. Sadly, therapeutic boarding schools can be costly. The average cost is

$4500 per month with a range of $2500 to $10,000 per month (Envoy Group, 2022).

Transitional Services

Billy is 21 years old. After high school he didn't really have a "life plan." He was working at a local car wash, but when his job was terminated for showing up late to work too many times, he didn't put in any applications at any other places of employment. Billy is comfortable living in his parents' home in the room he grew up in. He does his own laundry and makes his own meals, but he doesn't chip in with any of the other household chores, nor does he contribute to the family budget. This is not how his parents imagined Billy's life would be. They aren't sure what next steps to take.

Billy suffers from "failure to launch." Failure to launch has become increasingly more common in the last decade (Hendriksen, 2019). Young adults remain at home, comfortable with the idea of their parents taking care of them and not moving on after high school. This "Peter Pan Syndrome" is the phenomenon of adult children not making the transition to adulthood. *Transitional or independent living programs* for young adults provide a combination of therapeutic support and life skills training. Transitional programs may offer outpatient or residential treatment options. In addition to volunteering, the young adults are typically working part-time or taking a college course or two. These programs assist young people moving from adolescence to adulthood by supporting their independence.

When You Don't Know What Services are Needed

One of my children did not meet several of the above criteria. They were too stable to need "inpatient services" and facing crises not successfully being addressed by an IOP curriculum. We were at a loss.

My spouse and I wanted so much to see our child succeed, but we were not knowledgeable about resources available, let alone which program would be best. To best help our adolescent, we hired an educational and therapeutic consultant, commonly referred to as an EC.

Educational Consultant (EC)

Definition: A consultant who helps parents and students with educational and therapeutic planning. ECs are typically self-employed or employed by consulting firms.

Cost: EC fees can range between $85 and $200 an hour. Most clients purchase service packages which can range from $850 to $10,000 (College Planner Pro, 2022). The cost of an EC is generally not covered by insurance. If you are working with your EC specifically for therapeutic placement, you may be able to count a portion of the fees as a tax exemption, but I would discuss this on a case-by-case basis with your accountant.

How to Find Services: Unfortunately, I have discovered most therapeutic consultants are found by word of mouth. The Therapeutic Consulting Association does have a website that lists several members who offer placement services. Keep in mind that while an EC may not be located within your state, they may still be able to help you. Most ECs are familiar with programs across the nation.

Our EC recommended a therapeutic wilderness program for our teen. *Therapeutic wilderness* is an outdoor program that combines individual and group therapy with an experiential component. Although very challenging, these programs can be very nurturing and supportive. While our child participated in this program, they engaged in individual and group therapy, psychological evaluation, medication adjustment, while learning survival skills, completing high school credits, and learning self-care. As parents, we also had a curriculum to complete at home. We read books, attended parenting classes, learned self-care techniques, and became aware of how to better support our child.

Therapeutic wilderness programs are not cheap. A small portion of the cost can be submitted through your insurance provider, but frequently these programs are out-of-network and what is covered by insurance is only three hours of therapeutic care per day. In 2017, the average cost of these programs was $558 per day. An adolescent may be enrolled in a wilderness program for three to five months (Wilder, 2017).

How Do I Afford Behavioral Health Services?

Second to parents being frustrated by the lack of resources available in mental health for their child, I hear the cost of the services that are available may be more than the household budget allows. Over the years I have found parents will go above and beyond to invest in their child's mental health. When healthcare insurance does not cover the cost of treatment, I have observed parents taking out a low-interest equity loan from their bank or downsizing their home to afford treatment programs. Some individuals have had to sell vehicles or jewelry. Parents have cashed in bonds, stocks, an IRA or taken a 401K loan to make payments.

Often parents seek funding for treatment facilities through external sources. I have heard of parents asking family members, close friends, or their church for help. There have been GoFundMe pages started. Other individuals have gone to taking out behavioral health loans through Lightstream Medical Loans, Prosper Lending, M-Lend Financial, or Cross Bank Medical Financing (Envoy Group, 2022). If your child was adopted, funds may be available through Adoptive Families Coalition. In fact, California is required by state law to aid families with struggling adoptees who were once part of the California foster care system (Envoy Group, 2022). If your child was the victim of a crime, The National Association of Crime Victim Compensation Boards may be able to help you find resources to submit applications for funding (Envoy Group, 2022). On some social media pages, I have read about parents getting the local school district to fund some of the cost because the services needed for their child was more than the district could supply through an individualized educational program (IEP).

Wait? The School Can Help?

If a child's mental health is interfering with their performance at school, the child may qualify for an individualized education program (IEP). An IEP has two general purposes. First, an IEP should establish measurable annual goals for the child (Center for Parent Information & Resources, 2022). Second, the IEP should state the services the public agency will provide to, or on behalf of, the child. An IEP is a working document that allows for necessary accommodations as well as specially designed instruction. With an IEP, students can receive tailored instruction unique to their needs, goals, and objectives (Center for Parent Information & Resources, 2022).

Once a school system becomes aware of a child's needs, an academic assessment should be initiated. The school would contact the child's parents and, with parental consent, proceed with evaluating the child for service needs. Unfortunately, this is not always the case. If your school has not begun this process for your child or adolescent, and your child has been struggling academically due to their mental ailment, I recommend you reach out to the school's administrative team and formally request (I highly suggest in writing) an IEP evaluation. Once you have submitted a request for an IEP evaluation, the school district must respond within a given time frame. The allotted time for the school to respond is determined by each state (Lightner, 2022). In

Indiana, for instance, once the written request is made and the Permission to Evaluate has been signed, the school must assess the child and come up with a written IEP within 60 days. Some states have shortened this time frame to 30 or 45 days, but for most, it is 60 (Lightner, 2022).

Who Qualifies for an IEP? (Schmidt, 2022)

Autism	Blindness	Deafness	Emotional Disturbance
Hearing Impairment	Intellectual Disability	Multiple Disabilities	Orthopedics Impairment
Specific Learning Disability	Speech or Language Impairment	Traumatic Brain Injury	Visual Impairment

If your child does not qualify for an IEP, the school may suggest a 504. The purpose of a 504 Plan is to ensure that a child who has a disability identified under the law, and who is attending a primary or secondary educational institution, receives accommodations that will ensure their academic success (Schmidt, 2022). The difference between an IEP and a 504 is that an IEP provides specialized instruction for students. A 504 more commonly allows for student accommodations only (Schmidt, 2022). An IEP serves students in grades K-12, while a 504 plan can serve students in grades K-12 as well as college levels (Schmidt, 2022). Examples of accommodations in 504 plans include: preferential seating, extended time on tests and assignments, reduced homework, verbal or visual aids, modified textbooks, behavioral management support verbal testing, and adjusted class schedules.

Who Qualifies for a 504? (US Department of Education OCR, 2020).

Section 504 covers qualified students with disabilities who attend schools receiving Federal financial assistance. To be protected under a 504, a student must be determined to:

1. Have a physical or mental impairment that substantially limits one or more major life activities.

2. Have a record of such impairment.

3. Be regarded with such an impairment.

Note: A medical diagnosis is not needed to qualify for a 504 plan.

I have worked with families, both professionally and personally, that have children who qualify for an IEP or a 504 plan. I have reviewed educational plans with parents during medical visits to be sure the child has the resources in place to be successful. A child's mental health goes beyond the walls of the home. Academic success is important in a child's wellness. A child can spend 35 hours a week at school and how they perceive their environment and learn to adapt to the challenges they encounter is extremely important to their overall wellbeing. Unfortunately, some parents have found school resistance in starting an IEP or a 504 plan. If you feel your case is not being heard and additional resources are imperative for your child's success, consider consulting an educational attorney to find out what rights you and your child have.

Finding the right psychological services for your child may feel overwhelming.

The path for services is not well known by families. Unfortunately, understanding the variety and depth of resources available to individuals is also not well known to many frontline healthcare providers. The National Alliance of Mental Illness (NAMI) is a non-profit, voluntary health organization dedicated to providing mutual support, education, advocacy, and research funding for people affected by mental illness, their families, and friends. Many states have a local chapter. HelpLine volunteers are available to answer questions, offer support, and provide resources if you are struggling with the next steps. The NAMI HelpLine can be reached Monday through Friday, 10 a.m. – 10 p.m., ET. 1-800-950-NAMI (NAMI) or info@nami.org (NAMI, 2022).

Summary of Services: People

Primary Care Provider (PCP): A medical professional who may be both the first contact for an individual with an undiagnosed health concern, as well as providing continued care of varied medical conditions. For a child, this may be a pediatrician or a family medicine physician. PCPs may be a physician (MD, DO) or an advanced practice provider (NP, PA).

Behavioral Health Consultant (BHC): An individual who works with patients to address and improve behavior concerns.

Licensed Clinical Social Worker (LCSW): LCSWs assess, diagnose, and provide treatment for emotional and behavioral concerns. Many LCSWs provide outpatient counseling services.

Psychologist: A doctor who studies cognitive, emotional, and social processes and behavior by observing, interpreting, and recording how people relate to one another and to their environments. A psychologist cannot prescribe medication. Psychologists may have a degree as a PhD, PsyD, or EdS.

Psychiatrist: A medical professional who specializes in mental health and is qualified to assess medical conditions and prescribe medications.

Educational Consultant (EC): A consultant who helps parents and students with educational and therapeutic planning.

Summary of Services: Places

Outpatient: A patient who receives medical treatment without being admitted to a hospital.

Inpatient: A patient who stays in a hospital setting while under treatment.

Intensive Outpatient Services (IOP): IOPs are treatment programs used to address addictions, depression, eating disorders, or other dependencies that do not require detoxification or round-the-clock supervision.

Partial Hospitalization Services (PHP): While admitted to a PHP, the individual lives at home, but participates with behavioral health providers generally eight hours a day for five days a week, for two to four weeks, typically at a hospital setting.

Residential Services: A psychiatric residential treatment facility, or PRTF, is defined as a facility, other than a hospital, that provides live-in psychiatric services.

Transitional Services: *Transitional or independent living programs* for young adults provide a combination of therapeutic support and life skills training. Transitional programs may offer outpatient or residential treatment options.

Wilderness Services: *Therapeutic wilderness* is an outdoor program that combines individual and group therapy with an experiential component.

Homework: Keep a log of your healthcare providers for easy access.
(Additional Matter – Healthcare Team)

Chapter 4

PREPARING FOR YOUR FIRST MENTAL HEALTH VISIT

When I was in medical school, the professors spent a great deal of effort teaching the art of obtaining a detailed patient history. A patient's medical history includes information about past medical diagnoses, previous surgeries, current medications and supplements, allergies, and immunizations. It often contains health habits such as diet, exercise, and substances used (tobacco, alcohol, etc.) as well as medical conditions other family members have suffered. Clinical classes were required one or more times a week for an upwards of three hours to become proficient in patient interviewing skills. After our teachers believed we understood the basics, "practice patients" came to the school and each student was provided a minimum of thirty minutes to engage with the individual and learn about their history. Often, in those early academic training years, we would have an entire evening to put what we had learned into writing.

By the time I was in my third year of medical school, I was sent to work on various specialty rotations, often in a hospital setting. Medical students are generally the ones chosen to start the history taking process.

(If you have ever visited the hospital, you can identify the medical students by their short white lab coats, their smiling enthusiastic faces, and the quality time they spent with you writing down practically every word you said verbatim.) As a medical student, you have the luxury of balancing only a handful of patients that have been assigned to your care so that you will have time to learn about each case thoroughly. The medical student generally presents the information to their supervising team member (identified by the long white lab coat). In most cases this is an intern or resident. The resident takes the case to their supervising fellow physician. The fellow then informs the attending physician. (The attending physician is the person whose name most likely appeared on your hospital bill, but often the same physician you didn't see much during your stay.) This is how I was taught; then I graduated.

When you become the overseeing physician, the game changes. No longer do providers have the luxury of several hours to get a detailed medical history and lay out their therapeutic plan, but they are given a whopping 15 minutes, if they're lucky, to talk to the patient, generally about several topics, perform a detailed physical examination, order appropriate treatment, communicate the plan to the patient, answer any questions the patient may have, and then complete the required visit documentation. It's not that they suddenly feel they are too superior to take a thorough patient medical history or that they are not wanting to fully get to know their patient and spend time with them, it's just not how our current healthcare system has been operating. Sadly, most physicians see patients eight hours a day and then go home to spend another two or three hours working on chart documentation, attempting to submit prior authorizations for treatment plans to insurance companies, or responding to dozens of online patient inquiries about their current health status. According to Medscape's 2021 Physician Burnout Report, approximately 42% of current providers are struggling with mental health issues of their own based on the current healthcare system demands (Kane, 2021). (I suspect this number is under reported. In my experience physicians do not want to sound "weak" to themselves or others are not likely to admit it when they feel exhausted.) There are pockets of physicians trying to change this model of healthcare, but as a nation, we are not quite there yet.

So, you have an upcoming visit with your child's doctor to discuss your concerns about the child's mental health. How can you prepare for the visit? Great question! Let's enter your primary care provider's brain, shall we?

Step 1: Contacting the office to schedule an appointment.

At this point in the book, I'm sure you appreciate the complexity of mental health. While two children may share the same psychological diagnosis, they may present very differently depending on their age, environmental exposures, and genetic disposition. What is needed for treatment of one individual is not likely identical to what is needed for treatment of another individual. I recommend scheduling an appointment with your provider to discuss only the mental health issue for which you have concerns. (This is a great time to get out the highlighter! I'll give you a moment to highlight "an appointment with your provider to discuss only the mental health issue.")

As a physician, I frequently see children for their yearly well child check-up. During these visits, I spend time discussing the adolescent's physical state, I tackle concerns about where they are in social development, I complete their sports physical form, and I discuss what immunizations are due, if any. I end the visit with, "Is there anything else we didn't discuss today?" This is when I get bombarded by the "I think my child is depressed. Last week they told me they wish they were dead." Add the "dun-dun-dun" sound effect here.

At this point, I wish we would have spent the entire visit discussing this concern and rescheduled the well visit for another week. Depression, anxiety, or generally any other mental health ailment is easily a full appointment by itself. Now personally, I will never turn away a patient who tells me, at the moment my hand hits the doorknob and I'm saying goodbye, that they have additional mental health concerns.

I'm just strongly recommending making an appointment to fully address the topic up front.

If a mental health topic is a concern during an appointment, I will ask several questions. If the adolescent is over the age of 14, I will ask questions with both the child and their parent, and I will separate the child to another room and speak to them individually. I will ask about tobacco use, alcohol use, and illicit drug use. I will also ask about sexual activity. In many cases, I will provide one or two questionnaires for the child to complete so I can get a more complete picture of their day-to-day emotions. In my office I allow for a 30-minute appointment to talk to the child and their accompanying parent. In many offices, the provider is limited to 15 minutes.

As a parent, I appreciate how hard it is to take time off work, travel across town with multiple kids in tow, to get to the pediatrician's office on time with the insurance cards and the right kid for the right day of the right appointment. I understand that my child's provider has limited time; I, too, am a working parent with limited time. I appreciate that the doctor has a list of agenda items to complete for preventative care of my child; I also want to be sure to get all my agenda items discussed during the visit. So, is there a happy compromise to getting both my concerns for my child, and the doctor's concerns for my child, addressed in an efficient way? I'm so glad you asked! Before my child's visits I frequently write up a visit "itinerary." I provide my proposed list of items to discuss with the physician at the start of the visit, so they are aware of my concerns (I try to limit them to 3). I am understanding the topics may change based on the provider's suggested itinerary items (things I didn't think about). In some cases, a follow up appointment may be necessary to address everything.

Step 2: Creating an Itinerary
CC: ← This stands for "Chief Concern."

The chief concern is the main idea you want to discuss. For instance, "I think my child is depressed." This would be considered an itinerary item. In medical school we were taught to think very methodically. If you listen carefully after you announce an itinerary item, the follow up questions from your physician may follow a certain order. For mental health, it may look like this:

1. What was/were the precipitating factor(s)?

2. What is the extent of the condition?

3. What are the primary symptoms?

4. What is the duration of the symptoms?

5. Has the child ever had any concerns like this previously?

6. Has the child mentioned thoughts of harming themselves or someone else?

Having a brief outline of the chief concern and a few supporting details may help your provider allocate enough time during the visit to answer all your questions.

Step 3: Preparing Your Child's Medical History

Your child's medical history may look different depending on whether you are visiting your primary care provider or a psychologist doing a full mental health evaluation. In my family medicine office, I often want to know the following details:

1. Previous medical history:

    a. What illness has the child experienced?

    b. Has the child previously spent a night in the hospital?

c. Has the child ever fallen behind in meeting their developmental milestones and needed extra services such as physical therapy, occupational therapy, speech therapy?

2. Previous surgical history: It is helpful to know what procedure was done and when it was done when possible.

3. Current medications: This includes all supplements, vitamins, herbs, home remedies and over-the-counter medications.

4. Allergies: I am interested in both medication as well as environmental and food allergies.

5. Social History:

    a. Who does the child live with?

    b. Where does the child go to school?

    c. Does the child get along with others their age?

    d. Has the child had disciplinary issues at home? At school?

    e. Has the child experimented with tobacco, alcohol, or illicit drugs?

6. Sexual History

    a. Is the child sexually active? If yes, at what age did they become sexually active?

    b. What gender does the child identify with?

    c. Does the child identify with a specific sexual orientation?

7. Family History: I love to get as much family history as possible, but I am generally most concerned with the physical and mental health of the parents, siblings, aunts/uncles and grandparents. If there is a family history of mental illness, knowing what

medications parents and siblings have been successful on is often helpful.

8. Immunization History: Is the child up to date on vaccinations?

9. Anything else? For mental health, this may include names of previous counselors or psychiatrists. If the child was hospitalized, knowing where and when can help in obtaining past records. If the child has been on medications, knowing names of medication, dosing, when the medication was taken, and if appropriate, why it was stopped helps fill in the details of the child's story.

If your child has been established with your primary care provider for some time, the medical history is likely already up to date in the electronic medical record. If this is the first time your child is seeing a provider, or if you are unsure if there is missing information, writing out the medical history before the visit can save a great deal of time.

From my experience with my children, if you are visiting a psychologist the medical history may look a little different. I have completed many forms that look back to prenatal history. Questions I have previously been asked:

1. What was the prenatal home environment like? Was the mother abused physically, sexually, or emotionally?

2. Did the mother use tobacco, alcohol, or illicit drugs during the pregnancy?

3. Did the mother use other substances such as medications, supplements, herbs or caffeine, during the pregnancy?

4. Did the mother have any medical conditions identified at the time of pregnancy that caused complication to the pregnancy?

5. How long was the mother in labor?

6. Were there any complications with the delivery of the child?

7. How long did the child stay in the hospital before being released home?

8. Was the child fed breastmilk or formula?

The questions generally progress into early childhood development:

1. Who was the primary caretaker for the child during their first year of life? Second year of life?

2. Did the child meet their developmental milestones on time? If not, did they receive physical therapy, occupational therapy, or speech therapy?

3. How did the child interact with other children of a similar age?

4. Was the child frequently ill?

The more information about your child's history you can offer to a mental health provider, the more accurate the diagnosis. A correct diagnosis is critical to your child's success through treatment.

Remember Ryan from chapter one? I would like to take the time to show you what Ryan's itinerary may have looked like as his parents took him to the stress center that cool October evening.

CC (Chief Concern): Agitation and Physical Violence

History of Events:

Ryan is a 10-year-old male who had been watching YouTube with his brother. He became frustrated with his sibling and was unable to be redirected. Ryan's parents endured physical violence from Ryan. He was noted to push, hit, kick, and bite them. Ryan was unwilling to go to the stress center for an evaluation of a sudden change in behavior with his inability to emotionally regulate. The Crisis Intervention Team was called to help get Ryan safely to the stress center for intake. Ryan became calm when he saw the police officers and got into the vehicle for transport. Ryan has a history of anxiety and depression. He has had other episodes of violence in the past, but the recent episode was different in the duration and intensity of his outburst. The meltdown lasted over an hour before the Crisis Team was contacted.

You may recall the "provider follow up questions" I mentioned earlier. As you can see, we've addressed each of them.

1. What was/were the precipitating factor(s)?

    a. After watching television with his sibling, Ryan became frustrated by his brother's behavior.

2. What is the extent of the condition?

    a. Ryan became physically aggressive, especially towards his parents.

    b. Ryan did not have the ability to emotionally regulate and calm himself down.

3. What are the primary symptoms?

    a. Ryan was being physically violent.

4. What is the duration of the symptoms?

    a. Ryan was violent for more than an hour.

5. Has the child ever had any concerns like this previously?

    a. Ryan has a history of anxiety and depression that has led to previous outbursts.

6. Has the child mentioned thoughts of harming themselves or someone else?

    a. Ryan did not mention self-harm but was causing physical harm to others which prompted the urgent evaluation.

Ryan's Medical History

Ryan had not been seen previously at the stress center. The facility did not have a copy of his electronic medical record from his pediatrician. I strongly recommend creating a digital copy of your child's medical history. I have found this helpful to print before any new provider appointments, or to carry with me in case of an emergency visitation to a new location. An example may be as follows:

Ryan Smith

Date of Birth: March 27, 2009

Past medical history: No previous hospital stays.

Previous delayed milestone: Speech, received speech therapy for 3 years.

Past surgical history:

Circumcision, age 3 days.

Tonsils removed, age 3 years.

Current medications:

Multivitamin, one tablet once daily in the morning

Zoloft 100mg daily at night

Intuniv 1mg daily at night

Allergies: No known drug allergies.

Has anaphylaxis with bee stings.

Social history:

Ryan lives with his mother and father. He has three siblings in the home.

Ryan attends Lincoln Elementary School. He has two close friends.

Ryan does well at school but is frequently frustrated at home by his sibling. He does not handle changes to routine well.

Ryan has no history of tobacco, alcohol, or illicit drug use.

Sexual history:

Ryan is not sexually active. He identifies as a male.

Family History:

Mother: Anxiety, Obesity

Father: High cholesterol, Heartburn

Brother: Anxiety

Sister: No known health concerns

Maternal grandmother: Anxiety

Maternal grandfather: High blood pressure, Obesity

Paternal grandfather: Depression, Diabetes

Paternal grandmother: No known health concerns

Immunization history: Ryan is up to date on all childhood vaccinations for his age.

Current health care professionals:

Mary Jones, M.D.Pediatrician

1234 South Street, Avon, IN

(317) 555-1234

Paul Johns, LCSWCounselor

9876 East Street, Avon, IN

(317) 555-9876

Ryan's parents likely would not have had an "itinerary" to present to the stress center other than, "What is needed acutely to keep my child and the other children in the home safe?"

Let's look at home to prepare information for a psychological evaluation. For this I'm going to draw upon Jennifer's experience.

CC (Chief Concern): Depression, Defiance

History of Current Events:

Jennifer is a 14-year-old female who recently started high school. Prior to the start of the academic year, she was disheartened to find out her childhood friend was moving away. Fortunately, she was able to rekindle a relationship with another girl she knew from her time in gymnastics. Jennifer's new friend introduced her to a peer group with a different value system than she had previously demonstrated. Under the influence of these new adolescents, Jennifer started experimenting with drugs and sexual activity, skipping school, and stealing property. On one occasion she snuck out of her parent's home and participated in drinking and driving.

1. What was/were the precipitating factor(s)?

   a. Jennifer's friend moved away, and she felt lonely.
   b. Jennifer wanted to be liked by her new peer group.

2. What is the extent of the condition?

   a. Jennifer has participated in illegal activities.
   b. Jennifer has engaged in risky behaviors.
   c. Despite counseling and medication management, Jennifer's behaviors have continued.

3. What are the primary symptoms?

   a. Jennifer is defiant and ignores rules.

    b.   Jennifer is not eating. She has poor hygiene and sleeps several hours a day.

4. What is the duration of the symptoms?

    a.   Jennifer's behavior has worsened over the last few months.

5. Has the child ever had any concerns like this previously?

    a.   Jennifer's parents described her as an "easy child," prior to high school.

6. Has the child mentioned thoughts of harming themselves or someone else?

    a.   Jennifer has not mentioned thoughts of suicide or desiring harm to others.

Jennifer's Medical History

Jennifer Brown

Date of Birth: July 18, 2006

Past medical history: No previous hospital stays. No previous illness.

Jennifer's parents were married at the time of conception. Both the mother's pregnancy and delivery were without complications. The labor was approximately eight hours. Jennifer was born at 38 weeks' gestation. The mother did not use any tobacco, alcohol, or illicit drugs during the pregnancy. Jennifer went home from the hospital two days after birth. Her mother nursed her until she was one year old. Both Jennifer's mother and father played an important role in caring for her during her early years.

Jennifer met all her developmental milestones while growing up. She interacted well with other children. She was typically a physically healthy child.

Past surgical history: No previous surgical procedures.

Current medications: Lamictal 100mg each morning.

Allergies: No known drug allergies.

Will develop hives from peanuts.

Social history:

Jennifer lives with her mother and father. She has one brother and two half-sisters in the home.

Jennifer attends Greenstown High School.

Jennifer was previously an honor roll student. Since the change in her behavior, she is failing several classes.

Jennifer has no history of tobacco. She has experimented with alcohol and marijuana but denies chronic use.

Sexual history:

Jennifer has had one sexual encounter. She identifies as a female.

Family History:

Mother: Anxiety, Depression

Father: Diabetes, Hypertension

Brother: Anxiety

Half-Sister: No known health concerns

Half-Sister: Asthma

Maternal grandmother: Unknown

Maternal grandfather: Unknown

Paternal grandfather: Diabetes, Hypertension

Paternal grandmother: Breast cancer

Immunization history: Jennifer is not up to date on her childhood vaccinations. Her parents have opted out of vaccines secondary to religious preference.

Current health care professionals:

Mary Brown, M.D. Pediatrician

1234 South Street, Greenstown, IN

(317) 555-1234

Jeremey Miller, Ph.D. Psychiatry

4321 North Street, Greenstown, IN

(317) 555-4321

Rebecca Pearson, LCSW Counselor

9876 East Street, Greenstown, IN

(317) 555-9876

Itinerary:

What is the appropriate diagnosis for Jennifer's condition?

What is the treatment plan based on Jennifer's diagnosis?

What are the best resources to help facilitate Jennifer's treatment plan?

The more information available to the healthcare provider at the front of the appointment, the more productive you may find the visit. There is such a thing a thing as "too much information." What I have laid out is an example of a well-organized history which highlights the current events and medical background for very specific appointments.

Psychologists doing a full evaluation will welcome all past medical documentation from pediatrics, psychologists, social workers, schoolteachers, psychiatrists, etc. The more information provided, the better the specialist can evaluate your child. In my Family Medicine clinic, if I receive too much information during the appointment, I may not be able to get through it all and give you an answer before the end of the scheduled visit. I may request time to go back through it and devise a plan and call you with recommendations at a later date. Providing information to me, as a primary care physician, a week before the appointment would be best. If this is not possible, keeping a complete, but concise list of necessary information with highlighted points helps me when formulating a treatment plan.

Homework: Prepare for your child's first mental health visit (Additional Matter – Mental Health Visit Preparation).

Chapter 5

YOUR CHILD'S DIAGNOSIS

I t's Monday morning at the office. I've had my second cup of coffee and I am ready to go. My first patient is a ten-year-old male I have had the pleasure of caring for the past several years.

"Good morning!" I say as I walk through the door. I greet my patient and his mother and make my way to the stool near the room's computer. My patient's mother continues the conversation.

"Nicholas isn't listening to me. I tell him to pick up his room, nothing! I tell him to do his homework, nothing! When I tell him to get into the shower, he says no! He is very defiant, and I need medication that will help him."

I have seen this scenario all too often. Parents come to me asking for behavioral assistance with their child hoping for an easy solution. Unfortunately, there is no quick answer. Frequently a great deal of behavioral and even physiological work-up is needed to understand the complexities of the environmental and genetic situations affecting the adolescent. The "diagnosis" is not straightforward. So, I put on my doctor hat. "Can you tell me more?"

Nicholas' mother continues. "It started to get bad when he was in second grade. I would ask him to help me clean off the table after dinner and while he would do so, he complained the entire time. Now that he's in fourth grade, if I make a request he doesn't like, he immediately says no or agrees to complete the task, but never finishes it. I have tried taking away his cell phone. I have tried limiting his time with friends. I have tried having him write sentences about his behavior, but nothing ever works. If he does complete the punishment the same things that led to the consequence occur a few days later." I could see Nicholas' mother's exhaustion from caring for her son. Her intentions to have Nicholas' participation in chores and homework were good, however it was clear the current parenting strategy was not working.

I, too, have felt the sense of helplessness that comes when your child is struggling and you're not sure the right way to encourage them. The child is unsure how to feel better and yet they are unwilling for you as their parent to offer advice. Clearly what is occurring is not working for them, or for you. How is a parent to engage with a child who has checked out? How are they to support the child with no motivation to change? I remember my own parents telling me, "It takes a village to raise a child." I did not know what that meant until I had children of my own. Having a child struggling with behavioral issues may take a few skilled individuals to assist the child as well as his or her parents. If the child has special needs, it likely requires an entire care team of trained professionals.

Our home has five adolescents. Each teenager has their own challenges. My spouse and I have had to learn how to individualize our parenting approach for each one of them. No two kids fit the same mold. From the minute my child entered this world, they had a unique reaction to their environmental surroundings. Their experiences left an impression on them and created personal characteristics. One of the toughest things as a parent is believing I have finally found an approach that is effective for one of my kids only to find out it is completely ineffective for their sibling.

All is not lost. There are patterns to certain experiences siblings have in common and similarities to how teens with various diagnoses respond to therapeutic interventions. The trick is to be observant of your child, frequently ask them questions about their perceptions of an event and be prepared to change direction if the parenting course does not seem to be working for you or your child.

Medication management is sometimes a possible treatment option for children struggling with behavioral ailments such as inattention, low motivation, aggression, impulsivity, or other disrupting conditions. There are often integrative supplements, dietary support, and behavioral approaches also available in helping a youngster achieve wellness. Before treatment may begin, it is crucial to understand the underlying factors manifesting as behavioral challenges. The identification of the nature of an illness by examining its symptoms is known as a diagnosis (Google, 2022). A diagnosis is used to direct the child's care.

The Diagnostic and Statistical Manual of Mental Disorders (DSM-V) is a diagnostic tool published by the American Psychiatric Association. Essentially, it is a handbook for the assessment and diagnosis of mental disorders. The DSM-V does not contain treatment guidelines for the disorders found within its pages. Nevertheless, determining an accurate diagnosis is generally the first step in successful intervention of mental health conditions.

The DSM-V can be overwhelming. There are hundreds of disorders fully described by three major components: the diagnostic classification, the diagnostic criteria set, and the descriptive text. When my child was having behavioral challenges, my first instinct as a physician was to dive into the DSM-V to "get to the bottom of things." After all, if there was a diagnosis, there was a treatment. For example, if my child was "depressed" I assumed their pediatrician could prescribe a medication that would boost their serotonin levels (happy brain chemicals) and a licensed clinical therapist could meet with them to help them work through the events that led to their sadness. It sounded simple enough, right?

I have since learned teenagers with mood related concerns are medical marvels. Some teens follow Newton's third law of physics: when two bodies interact, they apply forces to one another that are equal in magnitude and opposite in direction. In parenting terms for those who have a child with mental health concerns, if a parent encourages an adolescent with mental health struggles to seek wellness, the child may meet them with an equal and opposite force of resistance to change. This can feel very defeating. I have found understanding my child's diagnosis has aided me to feel empowered to help them succeed by having a better understanding of their perspective. Having learned about my child's diagnosis and general patterns of behavior, when there is a decline in treatment success, I feel I have more patience and grace with my child than I had previously.

The top youth diagnoses can be divided into four categories: anxiety, mood disorders, Attention-Deficit/Hyperactivity Disorder, and disruptive behaviors. Anxiety, the first grouping, can be broken down into generalized anxiety disorder, social anxiety, panic disorder, panic attack, obsessive compulsive disorder, and post-traumatic stress disorder. Mood disorders include adjustment disorder with depressed mood, major depressive disorder, bipolar, and premenstrual dysphoric disorder. Attention-Deficit/Hyperactivity Disorder (ADHD) is an official medical condition, regardless of whether a patient demonstrates symptoms of hyperactivity. There are three types of ADHD: ADHD predominantly inattentive, ADHD predominately hyperactive, and ADHD combined both inattentive and hyperactive. Disruptive disorders contain oppositional defiant disorder and conduct disorder. Some individuals may have more than one diagnosis.

A: Anxiety Disorders

The most frequent diagnosis I treat in children, adolescents, and young adults is anxiety. I believe anxiety in this age group is easier to identify than other mental health ailments. Parents schedule appointments with me when their child is expressing overwhelming fear that is interfering with events at home and school. Anxiety can be paralyzing. Children may express they feel their heart racing, they cannot breathe, or they cannot focus. Children may be in constant motion during periods of increased anxiety. They may pace within a room or fidget excessively. Adolescents may be more irritable and react impulsively.

Generalized Anxiety Disorder and Social Anxiety

Jackie is a 19-year-old established patient in my medical clinic. For the most part, she is physically healthy. Her blood pressure on yearly physicals has been in the upper limits of normal, she has not been as active with exercise as ideal, and she has been noted as slightly overweight. Jackie, however, is not diabetic, her cholesterol is well controlled, she has no history of tobacco or alcohol misuse, and she does not require medication management. When Jackie turned 18-years-old, she went from living at home full time and having her parents support her financially, educationally, and socially to living in a college dorm funded by student loans, without anyone to check up on her studies, and surrounded by students excited to be "on their own" without parent curfews and rules. Jackie no longer felt the security she once did. She was unable to balance her finances. More than once, Jackie spent too much money on groceries and fun campus activities forgetting about laundry fees and bus fare to classes. Her grades declined because she would forget to turn in assignments. Jackie worried about not getting a job after college. She believed everyone knew how bad she was doing in her studies. She started skipping classes fearful everyone was watching her and going to insult her if she dared to attend lecture. Jackie began withdrawing from friends. She wouldn't answer her parents' phone calls. Her thoughts of failure preoccupied her to a point where she became unable to accomplish even the smallest task, such as showering.

The hallmark of generalized anxiety disorder (GAD) is excessive, out-of-control worry about everyday life events (Locke et. al, 2015). In GAD there may not be one single stressor. Individuals with GAD may suffer from several fears at once; and the trigger is not necessarily readily identifiable (Locke et. al, 2015). The worrisome thoughts interfere with daily functioning. Individuals with anxiety may present with physical ailments such as sleep troubles, fatigue, impaired concentration, irritability, muscle tension, or digestive issues (Locke et. al, 2015). The etiology of GAD is not well understood. Twin studies suggest both environmental as well as genetic factors may contribute. Research on GAD reports those who suffer more frequently from GAD include unmarried females, generally with lower educational levels, and the presence of life stressors (Locke et. al, 2015).

The DSM-V describes diagnostic criteria for GAD. In part, the DSM-V stipulates individuals may qualify for a diagnosis of GAD if they have excessive worry about several events over a period of six months (American Psychiatric Association, 2013). GAD may significantly impair an individual's ability to function at home or school. Often GAD is observed in social situations. To be declared GAD, the disturbance cannot be attributed to a medical condition, substance (such as a medication), or another mental health disorder (American Psychiatric Association, 2013).

Several scales are available to screen for GAD. The scale I use with patients in my office is the GAD-7. The GAD-7 has been validated to screen for anxiety and assess the severity of the individual's symptoms. (Locke et. al, 2015). The greater the GAD-7 score, the more functional impairment to one's life. To complete the GAD-7 questionnaire, an individual thinks about their thoughts over the previous two weeks and answers whether they felt this way "not at all," "several days," "more than half of the days," or "nearly every day." Each answer is scored with zero to three points. The scores of all seven questions are then added together for a final score. The final score helps determine if the individual has no anxiety, mild anxiety, moderate anxiety, or severe anxiety.

When evaluating a patient for an anxiety disorder, I look at possible physiological causes in addition to psychological ones. Endocrine conditions that impair thyroid function or adrenal gland tumors can cause sweating, increased blood pressure and rapid heartbeat (Locke et. al, 2015). Cardiovascular dysfunctions that cause abnormal heart rhythms or pulmonary ailments that cause shortness of breath may be mistaken as an episode of worry in an adolescent (Locke et. al, 2015). Children prone to seizures that affect the temporal lobe of the brain may present with signs of unexplainable fear (Locke et. al, 2015). In addition, certain prescribed medications such as albuterol for asthma and levothyroxine for thyroid disorder, or over the counter medications such as decongestants may produce feelings of uneasiness.

The standard American diet contains a great deal of processed sugars. Sugar increases dopamine (a messenger in the brain that drives behavior towards pleasurable goals) in the body (Greenblatt & Ross-Taylor, 2019). Dopamine helps the body maintain an enjoyable state and a sense of calm. When the body gets too much sugar, dopamine becomes excessive. The body attempts to regulate the influx by reducing the number of dopamine receptors (chemical catchers) in the brain (Greenblatt & Ross-Taylor, 2019). When the level of sugar reduces, there is not enough dopamine produced by the body alone due to the lower number of receptors now available. The individual starts to feel "withdrawal." Withdrawal symptoms can include trembling, increased thought patterns, heart racing and sweating (Greenblatt & Ross-Taylor, 2019). To relieve the symptoms, an individual feeds the body sugar unknowingly, causing the vicious cycle to continue, but removing the anxious feelings temporarily.

Unlike GAD which does not have a specific trigger, social anxiety disorder is activated by thoughts of an individual engaging with others or events an individual encounters with others.

When Kurt turned 21-years-old, he was excited to be able to go out to the bars with his friends. Kurt's friends were a few months older than he was and he was the last in the group to be included in the Friday night club entertainment. On the weekend following Kurt's birthday, Kurt's friend, Brad, asked Kurt to join him for a few drinks and some pool at the neighborhood bar. Kurt was excited to finally be included. As Kurt began to get ready for the evening out, he started feeling stressed. His hands started to sweat, his heart raced, and his stomach was tied up in knots. Kurt was worried about unknown aspects of the night. He didn't know what clothes to wear. He was unsure what the expectations at the bar would be like. He worried he didn't know what to ask for when his friends ordered drinks. Kurt worked himself up into a frazzled mess. An hour before Kurt was to meet Brad, Kurt changed his plans claiming he was ill and needed to stay home and rest. Kurt found it easier to hide at home than face an unknown situation around other people.

Social anxiety may include several forms of interpersonal interactions or experiences. I have had patients with concerns of social anxiety when it came to collaborating on projects, emailing a teacher, or ordering a pizza. In my professional experience with children and adolescents, I have seen more social anxiety in the past five to ten years. In some ways, I believe social media has placed a barrier to communication in front of our younger generation. Before posting to Twitter, Instagram, Snapchat, or TikTok teens can filter their thoughts and pictures. Conversations outside of the online world occur in real-time and without the ability to edit. Some adolescents may find this intimidating and struggle with communication skills.

It is normal to feel uneasy about a social event here or there. The hallmark of being diagnosed with social anxiety disorder is that an individual must exhibit symptoms of fear within multiple social settings for at least six months (American Psychiatric Association, 2013). The situation must also provoke feelings of worry that the individual will be judged negatively or embarrassed in these situations.

Anxiety – Panic Disorder and Panic Attack

Other forms of anxiety are Panic Disorder (PD) or Panic Attacks (PA). PD is characterized by recurrent and unexpected panic attacks. PA are isolated fearful events, typically peaking within ten minutes of onset and lasting several hours (Locke et. al, 2015). Many individuals have felt "panic" at some point in their lives. When fear of a situation overwhelms a person they may experience physical symptoms of sweating, dizziness, heart palpitations, difficulty breathing, numbness or an upset stomach. Their mind may race from one irrational thought to another, further escalating their response. PA may occur with another diagnosis, such as generalized anxiety disorder, social anxiety disorder, post-traumatic stress disorder, and agoraphobia. When the response occurs repetitively, and without a known trigger, a diagnosis of PD may be appropriate (Locke et. al, 2015). Individuals with PD may have a fear of losing control. Some individuals demonstrate feelings of "unreality" or "being detached from oneself" (American Psychiatric Association, 2013). Not all panic attacks have an unknown cause. An individual may feel panic in a specific situation, such as a speech in front of the class, seeing a spider, or trying out for a sport. Frequently, individuals with PD spend time modifying their behavior in maladaptive ways to avoid the possibility of a known trigger (American Psychiatric Association, 2013).

Kelly is a 13-year-old who is afraid of failing tests at school. Today Kelly's math teacher provided the class with a pop quiz. When Kelly starts to take the examination, her hands become clammy, and she starts to feel discomfort in her chest. Kelly struggles to focus on the questions and her leg starts to shake as she begins thinking about how the poor grade on the test may cause her to be ineligible to play softball next week. She notices her vision gets a little blurry and she feels dizzy. School examinations frequently lead to Kelly suffering from panic attacks. This is not the first time Kelly has done poorly on a test at school and didn't complete the assignment because of a panic attack. Later in the day Kelly thinks about ways to avoid having to go to school in the future so that she does not have to take any more exams. She starts to plan the illness she will use to stay home and miss next Monday's history test.

The DSM-V describes diagnostic criteria for PD. In part, the DSM-V stipulates individuals may qualify for a diagnosis of PD if they have recurrent and unexpected panic attacks. A panic attack is a sudden surge of fear. Physical sensations of panic attacks can include increased heart rate, sweating, difficulty breathing, shaking, trouble swallowing, chest discomfort, nausea, abdominal pain, dizziness, and numbness. Emotional disturbance during a panic attack may include fear of losing control, feeling detached, or feeling as though the individual is dying. In consideration for a diagnosis of PD, individuals demonstrate maladaptive changes in behavior, for at least one month, in hopes of avoiding a panic attack. To be declared PD, the disturbance cannot be attributed to a medical condition, substance (such as a medication), or another mental health disorder.

Anxiety – Obsessive Compulsive Disorder

Obsessive Compulsive Disorder (OCD) is characterized by frequent disturbing thoughts and repetitive behaviors or mental rituals to relieve a state of worry (Fenske & Petersen, 2015). Individuals with OCD may feel a sense of shame. They may complete their behaviors in secret to avoid criticism from others (Fenske & Petersen, 2015). In my medical practice, it's generally a family member or friend attending the appointment with a patient that brings up the maladaptive actions. Due to the "secret nature" of individuals with OCD, the diagnosis is generally not detected by providers early on. The age of onset for diagnosis is approximately 19 years old, however, it may be 11 years before they receive adequate treatment (Fenske & Petersen, 2015).

Scott couldn't sleep. He had been lying in bed for about ten minutes with the light off. He looked across the room where his computer sat on his desk. His eyes then darted to the night table. Scott stared at the lamp next to his bed. An alarm clock next to the lamp ticked away. Tick. Tock. Tick. Tock. Quickly Scott sat up and turned on the lamp. He moved to the desk and checked to be sure the computer cord was not plugged into the wall. He then walked to the night table and inspected the electrical outlet which powered the lamp and the alarm clock near his bed. The cords from the light and the clock did not touch. They lay across the floor, parallel to one another. Scott was very particular when it came to electrical cords, outlets, and the use of extension cords. When he was younger, he had seen a video on fire safety. Since the documentary, Scott checked, rechecked, and checked again the cords in his room before he went to bed to be sure there were no safety hazards.

OCD takes a toll on an individual's quality of life and overall functioning (Fenske & Petersen, 2015). Obsessions are repetitive, intrusive thoughts that cause individuals' distress. Thought patterns are unwanted by the individual and they take great effort to resist them. The thoughts may involve feelings of unworthiness, contamination, or be taboo in nature – such as is the case with thoughts of sexuality, aggression, or religion (Fenske & Petersen, 2015). Compulsions are behaviors that are repetitive or mental rituals that counteract the anxiousness provoked by an obsession. Frequent compulsions include seeking reassurance, handwashing, counting, checking, or praying (Fenske & Petersen, 2015). The DSM-V recognizes OCD distinctly from GAD.

The DSM-V describes diagnostic criteria for OCD. The DSM-V notes individuals may qualify for a diagnosis of OCD if they have obsessions, compulsions, or both (American Psychiatric Association, 2013). Individuals may attempt to suppress their anxiety by ignoring urges or fulfilling a particular task but are often unsuccessful. Obsessions and compulsions are often time-consuming and therefore interfere with plans to complete tasks at home and school. To be declared OCD, the disturbance cannot be attributed to a medical condition, substance (such as a medication), or another mental health disorder (American Psychiatric Association, 2013).

Anxiety – Post-traumatic Stress Disorder

Post-traumatic Stress Disorder (PTSD) has historically been identified in combat veterans, however, it is a relevant diagnosis for individuals who have been a victim to several other types of distressing situations (Warner et. al, 2013). The DSM-V characterizes PTSD by four general symptom domains: re-experiencing the event or intrusion symptoms; avoidance of people, places or things that serve as a reminder of the trauma; negative changes in mood and thoughts associated with the event; and chronic hyperarousal symptoms (American Psychiatric Association, 2013). Generally, the traumatic event involves a threat to one's life, one's sense of personal safety, or one's physical integrity (Warner et. al, 2013). PTSD can be differentiated from a similar condition, noted as Acute Stress Disorder, by the fact that PTSD persists beyond one month after the disturbing incident (American Psychiatric Association, 2013).

Both physical and emotional responses vary considerably in individuals who experience a traumatic stressor. Some individuals may not become symptomatic until several years after the incident (Warner et. al, 2013). When a person is unable to utilize adequate coping skills to process the trauma, psychological distress can intensify over time and lead to the development of PTSD. For this reason, early identification and treatment are important in improving prognosis. Self-report questionnaires can help providers in identifying anxiety associated with traumatic events. If I become aware of a patient experiencing a traumatic life event, I do my best to screen for PTSD. If the patient is not identified as having PTSD traits, ideally, they will be screened yearly thereafter to ensure timely intervention if needed. The Primary Care-Post-Traumatic Stress Disorder 5 (PC-PTSD-5) questionnaire can be used to quickly assess possible PTSD (Warner et. al, 2013).

Several co-morbid physical and mental health conditions can be associated with PTSD. Unless addressed properly, these additional ailments can adversely affect treatment. Common psychiatric comorbidities include anxiety, mood disorder (such as depression), and substance abuse. Common physical comorbidities include difficulty breathing, fatigue, headaches, muscle tension, pain, weakness, and elevated blood pressure (Warner et. al, 2013). Individuals with PTSD should be regularly screened for suicidal thoughts as one in five persons with PTSD may attempt self-harm. Physical injuries from a traumatic event increase the likelihood of PTSD (Warner et. al, 2013).

Daniel was excited to get his driver's license. He was officially 16 years old, and his parents had allowed him to borrow the family car to drive to his friend's house for the first time. Daniel spent the evening playing video games with his friend. By the time he was traveling home, it was late into the evening and already dark outside. Daniel took the country roads back to his house. He knew the roads were likely to have fewer cars on them than on the main streets through town. As Daniel came up to a curve in the road, he saw a deer jump out in front of him. Daniel was going too fast around the bend and in an attempt to miss the deer over-corrected and the vehicle ran off the road and head on into a tree. Daniel was shaken. He called his parents to come help. For several months after the accident Daniel refused to drive. Once he finally was able to get behind the wheel of a vehicle, he refused to drive at night. The thoughts of getting into an accident again would paralyze Daniel

and some days he would pull over onto the side of the road and call his
parents to drive him.

The DSM-V is very detailed in its diagnostic criteria for PTSD. Individuals may qualify for a diagnosis of PTSD if they have suffered an intrusive syndrome after being exposed to an actual or threatened injury, sexual violence, or death (American Psychiatric Association, 2013). The individual may have witnessed the event or been the victim. They may have learned of the encounter involving a close family member or friend (American Psychiatric Association, 2013). PTSD can also affect individuals who experience repeated or extreme exposure to details of a particular event. Intrusive syndromes that result after an incident are frequently manifested by recurrent and distressing memories or dreams (American Psychiatric Association, 2013). Individuals may have "flashbacks" in which they detach from their present self and feel as though they are reliving their past trauma. Many of the patients I have treated in my practice with PTSD have distinct physiological reactions to thoughts or to their environment as it resembles an aspect of the traumatic event.

Following trauma, individuals with PTSD often attempt to avoid the negative feelings they experienced by suppressing important details of the event (Warner et. al, 2013). Some individuals may blame themselves for the consequence of the trauma. Many victims suffer persistent fear, anger, guilt, or shame leading to estrangement from others. Traumatic events can cause marked alterations in arousal (Warner et. al, 2013). An individual's reactivity to a situation may include angry outbursts, recklessness, and hypervigilance. Individuals may struggle with concentration and impaired sleep. To be declared PTSD, the disturbance cannot be attributed to a medical condition, substance (such as a medication), or another mental health disorder (American Psychiatric Association, 2013).

Anxiety disorders can cause significant disruption not only in a child's life, but also within the family unit. When an adolescent is anxious they may be more irritable and respond negatively or aggressively to a simple remark such as "How was your day?" or "Will you please start your laundry?" Anxiety can reduce productivity causing longer times to complete homework. Anxiety may also reduce sleep quality or sleep duration leading to decreased mood, reduced motivation, and increased appetite. Fortunately, as we will see in the upcoming chapters, anxiety can be addressed through therapeutic intervention, dietary changes, nutritional supplementation, and if needed, medication management.

B: Mood Disorders

Mood disorders have many faces. While your child's situation is unique, you are likely to identify with a few patients I have treated recently.

Kristen is a 20-year-old who has been in therapy for the past three years. She has tried various medications, but she continues to have mood swings, especially before her menstrual cycles.

Mason is a 14-year-old whose depression worsened since starting high school. He has attempted suicide and been admitted into inpatient services as well as intensive outpatient services over the past year.

Ava is a 17-year-old with intense irritability and aggression. She refuses her medications because "they don't work" and will not talk in therapy because "they don't understand me!"

Nearly everyone has experienced depression at one time or another. Feeling sad and having little energy can occur after the loss of a relationship, missing a chance for advancement, or facing unwelcome change in your life. When the feelings become stronger and persist longer than what seems "normal," they can indicate a mood disorder. Mood disorders make it hard to function in day-to-day life. They can result in loss of relationships, loss of promotions, and affect physical health. Adolescents will generally describe their feelings as low energy, trouble sleeping, or unexplained pain rather than feeling "sad" or "depressed."

Major Depressive Disorder

Major depressive disorder (MDD) is one of the most common mental health conditions in the United States. The prevalence of depression is estimated at eight percent of those individuals older than the age of 12 (Maurer et. al, 2018). Globally, depression is the leading cause of disability, affecting more than 300 million people of all ages. The economic burden of MDD was estimated at $210.5 billion per year in 2018 (Maurer et. al, 2018). I suspect with the Covid-19 pandemic that number has increased significantly. If left untreated, depression may lead to suicide.

Risk factors for depression may come from internal factors, external factors, or adverse life events (Maurer et. al, 2018). Internal risk factors include females, history of anxiety, and low self-esteem. External risk factors include Conduct Disorder and substance abuse. Adverse life events include sexual abuse, chronic medical condition, disturbed family environment, parental divorce, parent loss, or low social support (Maurer et. al, 2018).

Symptoms of depression are commonly known by Sig E. Caps mnemonic.

S – sleep disorders (increased or decreased sleep patterns)

I – interest deficit

G – guilt (worthlessness, hopelessness, regret)

E – energy deficit

C – concentration deficit

A – appetite disorder (increased or decreased appetite)

P – psychomotor (agitation or lethargy)

S – suicidal thoughts

Depression may manifest differently between males and females. Women may report more physical ailments such as headaches, muscle aches and gastrointestinal symptoms (Maurer et. al, 2018). They are more likely to show emotional signs of stress such as crying. Men are more likely to report acts of aggression, anger, and substance use disorder or risky behaviors (Maurer et. al, 2018). This is not always the case, however.

The DSM-V describes diagnostic criteria for MDD. In part, the DSM-V instructs individuals may qualify for a diagnosis of MDD if they have depressed mood, reduced interest in activities they previously enjoyed, significant change in weight (gain or loss), alterations in sleep patterns (sleeps too much or too little), lack of energy, feelings of being a failure, decreased concentration, or recurrent suicidal thoughts (American Psychiatric Association, 2013). The symptoms cause distress at home and school. Socialization with others is impaired due to the individual's distress. To be declared MDD, the disturbance cannot be attributed to a medical condition, substance (such as a medication), or another mental health disorder (American Psychiatric Association, 2013).

The most widely used screening instrument for MDD in adolescents is the PHQ-9A (Maurer et. al, 2018). The PHQ-9A has been validated to not only to screen for depression, but also assess the severity of the individual's symptoms. The greater the PHQ-9A score, the more functional impairment to one's life. To complete the PHQ-9A questionnaire, an individual thinks about their thoughts over the previous two weeks and answers whether they felt this way "not at all," "several days," "more than half of the days," or "nearly every day." Each answer is scored with zero to three points. The scores of all seven questions are then added together for a final score. The final score helps determine if the individual has no depression, mild depression, moderate depression, or severe depression.

When evaluating a patient for a depressive disorder, it is important to look at both the physiological causes in addition to the psychological ones. Occasionally I'll need to order laboratory testing to ensure a physical cause may be excluded. A thyroid stimulating hormone test can help identify a thyroid condition. Thyroid disorder can cause fatigue and psychomotor changes. A complete blood count may be used to rule out anemia. Patients with anemia may have fatigue, depression, or weight loss. Pernicious anemia may cause mood changes or insomnia and warrant vitamin B12 testing.

Persistent Depressive Disorder (Dysthymia)

Liam is 13 years old. He spends most of his days after school lying in his bedroom in the dark. He doesn't come to the dinner table when food is served. He no longer asks to visit his friends. The symptoms started a year ago when he started middle school. He also struggles to concentrate on his schoolwork. When his parents ask him "What's wrong?" he grumpily says, "Nothing!" and walks away.

Persistent depressive disorder (PDD) (dysthymia) is a depressed mood, most of the day, for more days than not (Greenblatt & Lee, 2019). In children and adolescents, mood can be irritable, and the duration must be least one year. In PDD the decreased mood must present with at least two of the following: poor appetite or overeating, insomnia or hypersomnia, low energy or fatigue, low self-esteem, poor concentration, and feelings of hopelessness (Greenblatt & Lee, 2019). MDD may come before persistent depressive disorder and MDD episodes may occur during PDD. When PDD occurs before the age of 21-years-old, there is an increased likelihood of co-occurring personality disorders and substance use disorders (Greenblatt & Lee, 2019).

Disruptive Mood Dysregulation Disorder

Matt is 12 years old. His favorite pastime activity is watching Marvel movies on television. One weekend afternoon Matt sat in the living room in a recliner watching the newest Spiderman. His older brother, David, who was 14 at the time, came in and sat down on the sofa near Matt. David had already seen the movie.

"My favorite part is coming up!" David exclaimed.

"Don't tell me! I've been waiting to watch this all week," Matt replied.

"Watch this part. This is where…"

"Stop!" Matt interrupted his brother. "I don't want to know."

David had a bowl of chips in hand to snack on. Crunch! Matt could hear David munching on his snack nearby. "You're so loud!" Matt yelled and he put his fingers in his ears to block the sound. "Go away! I don't want you in here."

"You can't tell me where to go or what to watch Matt," David told him. With that David opened his mouth and took in a chip. He crunched as loud as he could to irritate his brother.

Matt got up from his chair, walked to David and used his foot to kick the bowl of chips David had been eating. He then started to grab David's t-shirt until David tackled him to the ground and pinned him. Matt tried to get back at David by attempting to bite David's arm.

Disruptive mood dysregulation disorder (DMDD) includes severe and persistent irritability. The child's conduct is more than what would be considered a "temperamental child." Children present with verbal and/or behavioral outbursts that are out of proportion in intensity or duration to the situation (Greenblatt & Lee, 2019). The outbursts are frequent, at least three or more times per week, over at least one year, and occurring in at least two settings (such as home and school) (American Psychiatric Association, 2013). The behaviors are developmentally inappropriate. When the child is not having an outburst, the child generally demonstrates persistent angry moods. This irritability is likely to occur most of the day, more days than not, and is noticeable by others (Greenblatt & Lee, 2019). The diagnosis is generally made in children ages six to 18. The initiation of disruptive moods must occur before the age of ten. There also may not be a period of greater than three months without the child demonstrating the above criteria (American Psychiatric Association, 2013).

As you can imagine, DMDD can have a significant impact on a child's family as well as peer relationships and academic performance. The threshold of frustration is extremely low for these children, and they may struggle participating in extracurricular activities generally enjoyed by other children (Greenblatt & Lee, 2019). They may also struggle to start and maintain friendships. Between two and five percent of adolescents are affected by DMDD (Greenblatt & Lee, 2019). DMDD is generally seen more in males and school age children than females and adolescents. Many children have other disorders, particularly oppositional defiant disorder, attention-deficit/hyperactivity disorder, or an anxiety disorder (Elia, 2021).

Premenstrual Dysphoric Disorder

Rachel has been struggling both physically and emotionally. Her stomach hurts. Her head hurts. She is extremely irritable. Her mother notices that every month over the past few years Rachel has had similar cycles. Just prior to Rachel's menstrual period she will have extreme fluctuations in her mood, she'll say she doesn't feel well, and she may even miss a few days of school. Rachel's symptoms return to "normal" a few days into her menstrual cycle. Rachel's mother understands Premenstrual Syndrome (PMS) can make you a little grumpy, but this seems way more severe than she's ever experienced.

Premenstrual disorders affect females of childbearing age. There are two premenstrual disorders, premenstrual syndrome (PMS) and premenstrual dysphoric disorder (PMDD). PMS and PMDD include mental and physical symptoms that develop within the last phase of a female's menstrual cycle and resolve shortly after menstrual bleeding begins (Hofmeister & Bodden, 2016). PMS and PMDD occur monthly. In PMS, the female suffers physical and emotional ailments, but she remains able to function in activities at home and school. PMDD is a much more severe form of PMS (Johns Hopkins Medicine, 2022). Females suffering from PMDD endure significant symptoms that makes it hard to function at home and at school. Both PMS and PMDD require attention and treatment. Lifestyle changes and sometimes medication management may be effective in helping an individual manage their symptoms (Johns Hopkins Medicine, 2022).

The DSM-V describes diagnostic criteria for PMDD. Females with a diagnosis of PMDD experience marked mood swings, irritability, feelings of hopelessness, or strong anxiousness starting in the final week before the onset of menses and improving shortly after the menstrual cycle begins (American Psychiatric Association, 2013). Females struggling with PMDD may lack interest in usual events. They report inattention, lack of energy, changes in appetite, and alterations in sleep patterns (American Psychiatric Association, 2013). These females frequently express they feel overwhelmed or out of control. Physical symptoms complicate emotional regulation further by creating sensations of swelling, muscle aches, breast pain, and bloating (Greenblatt & Lee, 2019). To be declared PMDD, the disturbance cannot be attributed to a medical condition, substance (such as a medication), or another mental health disorder. The symptoms are usually documented for at least two symptomatic menstrual cycles (American Psychiatric Association, 2013).

There is poor understanding of the etiology of premenstrual disorders (Johns Hopkins Medicine, 2022). Several studies suggest cyclical changes in estrogen and progesterone levels trigger symptoms. Many females report symptoms worsen as they approach menopause. Premenstrual disorders affect up to 12% of female (Hofmeister & Bodden, 2016).

Depression Induced by Substance Use or Medication

In substance use or medication induced depression, the symptoms of depressive disorder are noted, but they are associated with the ingestion of a substance (drug, alcohol, medication, or another toxin) (Greenblatt & Lee, 2019). Typically, the onset of reduced mood begins within the first few weeks of initiation of the substance. Once the substance is discontinued, the depressive symptoms begin to diminish. It may take a few days to several weeks for the mood to become stable depending on the substance that was utilized and whether the individual suffered withdrawal (Greenblatt & Lee, 2019). Substances that may mimic depression include alcohol, heroin, bath salts or other designer drugs. Prescribed medications that may mimic depression include isotretinoin (used for acne), oral contraceptives (birth control), high blood pressure medications, cholesterol medications, or medications used to treat depression and anxiety such as benzodiazepines (e.g., alprazolam (Xanax), temazepam (Restoril), diazepam (Valium), clonazepam (Klonopin) (Schimelpfening, 2020).

Depression Induced by Medical Illness

Jenny is in the eighth grade. About a month ago she started to feel tired, her muscles ached, and she had presented with a headache and sore throat. In fact, it hurt so much to swallow Jenny's parents fought with her to stay hydrated. Jenny's mother made an appointment with Jenny's pediatrician. Jenny was diagnosed with mononucleosis (mono for short). While Jenny has started to feel better, and has recently been able to return to school, she still feels exhausted all the time. The eighth-grade girls are about to start the rugby season. Jenny loves rugby. Her doctor has not yet signed off on Jenny's ability to return to sports. Jenny is frustrated. She doesn't feel well, she would rather stay in bed, and she feels isolated from her friends. When she gets home from school she heads to her room and sleeps. She has not desired interaction with others around her.

Physical ailments are known to influence mood (Greenblatt & Lee, 2019). When an individual faces a significant injury or infection, chemicals called cytokines signal the immune system to do its job. Cytokines control the growth and activity of immune system cells and blood cells to help with healing. Cytokines may increase neurotransmitter release in the process (Greenblatt & Lee, 2019). When the body sees increased neurotransmitters in the brain, it reduces previous neurotransmitter production (Greenblatt & Lee, 2019). When the supply of neurotransmitters is less than the demand for neurotransmitters, this can lead to depression or other mental illnesses.

There are several chronic conditions that are associated with depression. For instance, depression is the first psychiatric symptom of Huntington's Disease. Cushing's Disease and hypothyroid disorder are two other common conditions that have been closely tied to depression (Greenblatt & Lee, 2019). In children, I have observed infections such as mononucleosis, metabolic conditions such as insulin-dependent diabetes, respiratory conditions such as cystic fibrosis, and childhood cancers to cause children's mood to reduce based on their need for frequent healthcare visits and inability to participate in activities with their peers.

Depression with Anxious Distress

An individual may present with both depression and anxiety. These two conditions can even occur at the same time (Smith, 2021). When individuals experience anxiety, they may find it extraordinarily difficult to actively participate in treatment. Anxious distress may include feeling tense, unusually restless, poor concentration, fear that something awful will occur or that the individual may lose control (American Psychiatric Association, 2013). Individuals experiencing depression and anxious distress may isolate from others, consume themselves with negative thoughts, and suffer reoccurring feelings of sadness. The longer an individual remains in this hyperexcitable state, the more likely they will struggle to respond to treatment. High levels of anxiety increase an individual's risk for suicide (Greenblatt & Lee, 2019).

Depression with Atypical Features

Lucas was described by his peers in high school as a loner. He sat by himself at lunch. He turned down anyone who invited him to participate in after school activities. Lucas' grades were poor, not because he wasn't intelligent, he just wasn't motivated to do the work. Lucas wore his AirPods whenever he walked between his classes in hopes of avoiding conversations with others. One day in PE the class was playing basketball. Lucas enjoyed basketball and really got into the game. He was laughing and joking with his classmates for most of the period. Once class was over, Lucas returned to his AirPod wearing avoidant ways.

Atypical depression occurs when an individual meets the criteria for MDD, but also shows signs not usually associated with a depressive state. For instance, an individual may have MDD, but when their environment becomes more positive, their mood improves, even for a period, until either the positive environment changes, or the individual withdrawals from the environment to their previous state. This type of response is called mood reactivity (Greenblatt & Lee, 2019).

Other features of atypical depression may include weight gain, sleeping ten or more hours a day, leaden paralysis (feeling weighted down in the arms and/or legs), and sensitivity to rejection (Greenblatt & Lee, 2019).

Depression with Seasonal Pattern (Seasonal Affective Disorder)

It was early February. The clouds had been grey for a long time in northern Indiana. Temperatures averaged 20°F. There was one inch of frozen snow that covered the countryside, but even more ice below it.

Elizabeth laid in her bed. It was already late morning, but she didn't feel like getting up. Her friends had asked her to go out shopping today, but she didn't feel like being around others. Elizabeth wanted to sleep. She lacked motivation to begin the homework she had already fallen behind in. She thought back to the years prior. She hated winter. She always felt this way from December until early April when the flowers started to bud, and the sunshine started to warm the earth.

Seasonal affective disorder (SAD) is observed when the start of depressive episodes coincides with a particular time of year (Greenblatt & Lee, 2019). Symptoms of major depression that may occur seasonally include reduced energy, increased desire to sleep, increased appetite leading to weight gain, and a craving for carbohydrates. SAD has been linked to a biochemical imbalance in the brain caused by the shorter daylight hours (Greenblatt & Lee, 2019). For this reason, SAD is more common in individuals who live further from the equator where areas experience less hours of sunlight during the colder months. Younger adults and females are at higher risk for SAD. SAD may occur at any age, but the most common age of onset is between 18 and 30 years old (Greenblatt & Lee, 2019).

Bipolar Disorder

Rebecca's roommates were at a loss. A few weeks ago, Rebecca's boyfriend was killed in a motorcycle accident. He had been driving on a country road at night, with limited light availability, when he hit a deer and flipped his bike. Rebecca had not left the apartment since the incident other than to attend the funeral services. She laid on the sofa binge watching shows, ate very little, and spent several hours crying in the shower. This week however, there was a drastic change in Rebecca's behavior. It appeared she had decided to "move on." She was leaving the residence to party late into the night with people she had never previously mentioned. She was buying elaborate gifts for herself, like new Gucci sunglasses and a Louis Vuitton bag. When she was terminated from her job as a barista due to failure to show up to her shift, she didn't seem to mind. Rebecca rarely slept, yet she didn't seem tired, and her mood appeared to be overly happy. "Life's short! I might as well enjoy it!" she told her roommates.

Many individuals are surprised to find out there is more than one type of bipolar disorder. Bipolar disorders comprise recurrent episodes of elevated mood and depression (Marzani & Neff, 2021). Bipolar I includes mania, a distinct period of abnormally and persistently elevated, expansive, irritable mood with heightened energy, lasting at least one week and which is persistent most of the day. In contrast, Bipolar II consists of hypomania, a milder version of mania that lasts for a shorter period, usually a few days (Marzani & Neff, 2021). Rapid cycling, at least four mood episodes in the previous 12 months demarcated by partial or full remission for at least two months, or a switch to an episode of depression, can be applied to Bipolar I, but not Bipolar II (Marzani & Neff, 2021). Both Bipolar Type I and Type II may contain a period of depressed mood. Individuals typically present to my office requesting help for their reduced mood. The depression that is identified with bipolar is hard to distinguish from the unipolar (persistent feeling of sadness) depression. Patients do not typically present for care with hypomania. Despite negative consequences, hypomania creates a state of heightened mood and energy. This is often seen as desirable by the patient. When meeting with a healthcare provider, it is important to note whether your child has ever experienced manic behavior.

Bipolar disorders are multifactorial conditions (Marzani & Neff, 2021). Both genetic predisposition and environmental factors play a role in the development of the condition. Children of parents with bipolar have up to a 15% risk of inheriting the disorder (Marzani & Neff, 2021). While a child may be biologically susceptible to the ailment, it's typically stressful life events, trauma, death of a loved one, disordered sleep, or other physical processes that cause central and peripheral nervous system inflammation that can trigger the illness. For as many as 25% of patients with bipolar may present with a seasonal pattern (Marzani & Neff, 2021). Bipolar Disorders do not affect one specific race, sex, ethnicity, or socioeconomic status more than another. The mean age at onset is 18 years old in bipolar I and 22 years old in bipolar II (Marzani & Neff, 2021).

When considering a bipolar diagnosis, medical providers may first want to exclude physiological conditions. This is generally done through blood and urine testing. Typical blood work might contain an ammonia level (especially if the individual is taking seizure medication, such as valproic acid (Depakote), and presenting with mental status changes), a metabolic panel (to look at blood sugar, kidney, and liver function), a complete blood count (to rule out pernicious anemia), a lipid profile (cholesterol), thyroid stimulating hormone, urinalysis (to rule out infection), or urine toxicology screen (to look for substance use disorders) (Marzani & Neff, 2021). Imaging, such as an MRI of the brain, may also be ordered on a case specific basis.

Individuals diagnosed with bipolar are more likely to develop cardiovascular disease than those individuals in the general population (CardioSmart, 2015). They may also be at risk for metabolic conditions and need regular monitoring of blood sugar and cholesterol readings (CardioSmart, 2015). There are several reasons for this increased risk, including: unhealthy lifestyle choices, access to healthcare, and medication side effects. In addition, depression and stress have been linked to increased inflammation which is closely related to heart disease (CardioSmart, 2015).

The DSM-V describes diagnostic criteria for bipolar disorder. For a diagnosis of Bipolar I to exist, an individual must have suffered a manic episode (American Psychiatric Association, 2013). A manic episode is a distinct period when an individual has abnormal and persistently elevated mood and increased energy. The time the individual acts in this fashion is most of the day, nearly every day, for at least one week (American Psychiatric Association, 2013). In part, the DSM-V stipulates the individual may present with inflated self-esteem, decreased need for sleep, a pressure to keep talking, excessive distractibility, racing thoughts, and involvement in activities that may lead to unfortunate consequences (American Psychiatric Association, 2013). In Bipolar I, the episode is sufficiently severe to cause marked impairment in the person's life and hospitalization may be necessary in some cases to prevent harm to self or others (Marzani & Neff, 2021).

As discussed previously, not all individuals with bipolar disorder are deemed Bipolar I. An individual may meet the criteria for Bipolar II if their manic episodes are milder in presentation. Like Bipolar I, the individual with Bipolar II will present with elevated mood and increased energy. For Bipolar II, however, the time the individual acts in this fashion is most of the day, nearly every day, for a minimum of four consecutive days (American Psychiatric Association, 2013). The DSM-V notes the individual may present with inflated self-esteem, decreased need for sleep, a pressure to keep talking, excessive distractibility, racing thoughts, and involvement in activities that may lead to unfortunate consequences (American Psychiatric Association, 2013). In the case of Bipolar II, the episode is not severe enough to cause significant impairment in the person's life and the amount of change compared to when the individual is not symptomatic is unequivocal.

Whether classified as Bipolar I or Bipolar II, the individual is likely to face a major depressive episode. The DSM-V describes the depressive episode may present with decreased mood, reduced pleasure in activities previously enjoyed, change in weight, sleep disturbance, lack of energy, feelings of worthlessness, indecisiveness, and suicidal thoughts (American Psychiatric Association, 2013). The depressive symptoms of Bipolar II can be more severe and last longer than the depressive symptoms of Bipolar I (Marzani & Neff, 2021). Major depressive episodes impact an individual's ability to function. To be declared bipolar disorder, disturbances cannot be attributed to a medical condition, substance (such as a medication), or another mental health disorder (American Psychiatric Association, 2013).

Noah is 20 years old. He is majoring in pre-law and dreaming of someday being a corporate lawyer. Noah's academic schedule is very intense. Frequently he pulls all-nighters studying for upcoming examinations. His diet is poor as he is known to grab food on the fly out of the vending machine near his classes. Noah's exercise involves biking to lectures. Over the past two years, Noah's girlfriend has noticed fluctuations within Noah's behavior. During the spring and late fall Noah has periods of enhanced mood. He has increased energy, is able to stay up late – even for days in a row, is very talkative, showers her with gifts, and boasts of how his accomplishments will help him secure a spot in the best law school. There are other times during the year where Noah doesn't want to leave his apartment and turns down spending time with friends. He exhibits low self-esteem. While he can get his schoolwork done, he has little energy to do much more.

At first glance, Noah may appear to have bipolar disorder. He exhibits features of hypomania as well as depressive disorder. Noah actually suffers from a condition known as Cyclothymia. Cyclothymia is a milder variant of bipolar disorder. While moods are less intense, the highs and lows typically last longer. To make this diagnosis, the person usually has symptoms for at least two years (American Psychiatric Association, 2013). Individuals presenting with symptoms of cyclothymia are encouraged to work with a counselor to help develop emotional regulation skills and lifestyle choices which promote a better school/work/life balance.

In my clinic when I screen for bipolar disorders, I may use the Mood Disorder Questionnaire (MDQ). The MDQ is a one-page document which was developed and validated to screen for bipolar spectrum disorder (Hirschfeld et. al, 2000). The questions take less than five minutes to complete. Patients simply check the yes or no boxes in response to the questions. The last question helps assess the patient's level of functional impairment.

C: Attention-Deficit/Hyperactivity Disorder

I know of two brothers diagnosed by a medical professional with Attention-Deficit/Hyperactivity Disorder, or ADHD. Although they share the diagnosis, they present very differently. One of the brothers is very active and is always on the go. He moves from one place in the house to another looking for projects to do. His parents can generally tell where he's been because there are small piles of things he started, but didn't necessarily finish, along his path. His actions may be impulsive. For instance, he may cut a hole in the screen of his bedroom window to throw a paper airplane outside and see how it flies without thinking through the long-term effects of bugs climbing in his room at night or the fact his parents will be furious with a great big hole in the screen of a window they had recently replaced. The other brother can generally be found in one location. If left to his own desires, he would hang out in his bedroom all day. He must be reminded three times to take a shower, two times to get dressed, and a half dozen times to start his homework. When you talk to the second brother, he can talk without ceasing for an hour. His words come out as a string of thoughts. Unfortunately, "think before you say something you'll regret" is not at the forefront of his conversations with others. Two individuals, both lacking focus, but both very creative, passionate and intuitive in what interests them.

ADHD is not a behavioral problem, nor is it a problem with discipline. ADHD is a medical condition through which imbalances in the brain caused by genetic, neurological, nutritional, and environmental factors may have led to a behavior (Greenblatt & Gottlieb, 2017). ADHD is the most common neurodevelopmental condition affecting children in the United States (Chang et. al, 2020). An estimated 8.4% (greater than five million) children between the ages of two and 17 years of age currently struggle with ADHD. The average

age at ADHD diagnosis is seven years (Chang et. al, 2020). Boys are more commonly diagnosed than girls. Of those diagnosed, slightly more than 60% are treated with medication, less than 50% have received behavioral treatment, and approximately 25% have not received treatment at all (Chang et. al, 2020).

Children with ADHD are at risk for long term morbidities, such as poor academic performance, low self-esteem, difficult relationships, substance abuse, injury, or other maladaptive behaviors (Chang et. al, 2020). A parent should consider evaluation for ADHD by a mental health provider when there are concerns for a child's academic or behavior problems, including concerns of inattention, hyperactivity, or impulsivity at both home and school when a child is between four and 17 years of age. Diagnosing children four to six years of age is challenging because ADHD criteria may overlap with age-appropriate behaviors.

The DSM-V describes diagnostic criteria for ADHD. In part, the DSM-V expresses individuals may qualify for a diagnosis of ADHD if they experience a significant pattern of inattention and/or hyperactivity-impulsivity that interferes with function or development.

ADHD is typically specified as one of three diagnoses:

1. **Combined presentation**: If both inattention and hyperactivity-impulsivity are demonstrated for the previous six months.

2. **Predominately inattentive presentation**: If inattention is demonstrated, but hyperactivity-impulsivity is not demonstrated for the previous six months.

3. **Predominantly hyperactive-impulsive presentation**: If hyperactivity-impulsivity is demonstrated, but inattention is not demonstrated for the previous six months.

Symptoms of inattention may include failing to give close attention to details, difficulty sustaining focus in tasks, trouble following instructions, inability to maintain organization, avoidance of tasks that require persistent mental effort, frequent misplacement of things necessary for daily tasks, easy distractibility, and repetitive forgetfulness (American Psychiatric Association, 2013). When having a conversation with an individual who suffers inattention, they may appear as though they are not listening even when spoken to directly.

Symptoms of hyperactivity-impulsivity may include continuous fidgeting, difficulty remaining in seat in situations where it is expected, difficulty engaging in leisure activities quietly, frequently seen as "on the go," excessive talking, inability to wait one's turn, and frequent interruptions or intrusions on others (American Psychiatric Association, 2013).

To be diagnosed with ADHD, the DSM-V notes individuals should present with symptoms prior to the age of twelve. The symptoms should be present in two or more settings, such as home and school (American Psychiatric Association, 2013). There must be clear evidence inattention and/or hyperactivity-impulsivity reduces the individual's ability to function in their environment. The symptoms must also not be able to be explained by another mental disorder.

Several scales are available to screen for a diagnosis of ADHD. The scale I use with patients in my office is provided by the National Institute for Children's Health Quality (NICHQ) and is known as the Vanderbilt Assessment Scale. When a parent has concerns about their child's behavior, I provide the parent with a copy of the "Parent Assessment Scale" and the "Teacher Assessment Scale." The parent returns the evaluations to me to be scored and we schedule a telephone call or video visit to go over the results. What I like about the Vanderbilt Assessment is that it evaluates ADHD, as well as provides me insight as to whether I should look further into other mental health conditions such as oppositional defiant disorder, conduct disorder, anxiety, depression, or learning disabilities. Other screening tools for ADHD include Child and Adolescent Behavior Inventory, Child Behavior Checklist, Conners Comprehensive Behavior Rating Scales, Conners Early Childhood,

Brown ADD Rating Scales for Children, Adolescents, and Adults, ADHD Rating Scale, and Conners Third Edition (Chang et. al, 2020).

When evaluating a patient for ADHD, I look at possible physiological causes in addition to psychological ones. Possible physical conditions that may mimic, or co-exist, with ADHD include Fetal alcohol syndrome (FAS), genetics (e.g., fragile X, neurofibromatosis, or 22q11 deletion syndromes), hearing loss, neurological disorders (e.g., seizures, traumatic brain injury, Tourette syndrome, or other tic disorders), sleep disorders (e.g., insomnia, obstructive sleep apnea, restless leg syndrome, or periodic limb movement disorder), and musculoskeletal disorders (e.g., reduced motor coordination or unintentional injuries) (Chang et. al, 2020). Possible mental health ailments that may mimic, or co-exist, with ADHD include anxiety disorders, autism spectrum disorders, mood disorders, oppositional defiant disorder, conduct disorder, and substance use. Possible situational factors that may mimic, or co-exist, with ADHD include specific learning disabilities (e.g., reading, math, or writing), behavior (e.g., school suspensions or expulsion), home environment (such as survivor or child abuse), motivation (e.g., loss of motivation or learned helplessness), and psychosocial difficulties (e.g., bullying, peer rejections, adult disapproval, poor self-esteem, difficulty learning rules or understanding social cues). At least 60% of children with ADHD meet criteria for at least one other mood disorder (Chang et. al, 2020). Since these conditions may already exist, or emerge over time, parents and clinicians should work together and reassess the child regularly to be sure the best treatment intervention is being applied.

Treatment for ADHD may vary based on the age of the child. Parent training in behavioral management (PTBM) is typically recommended for parents of preschool to middle school children. PTBM addresses expectations of a child's behavior and works to strengthen parent-child relationships while supporting behavior change via positive reinforcement techniques (Chang et. al, 2020). PTBM can be taught to parents by a therapist in a private or group setting. PTBM is less likely to be effective if the parents of the child have differing expectations and commitment to the therapeutic approach. Alternative therapies such as mindfulness, cognitive behavioral therapy, supportive counseling, and use of cannabidiol oil have not shown significant benefit in patients with ADHD (Chang et. al, 2020). Therapeutic treatments will be further discussed in chapter 6.

Typical medications for the management of ADHD include stimulants. Nearly 90% of patients show benefits from this type of medication (Chang et. al, 2020). Non-stimulant medications that may be prescribed include atomoxetine (Strattera), extended release guanfacine (Intuniv), and clonidine. Unfortunately, there are not any available pharmacological tools or symptom checklists to guide appropriate choice of which stimulant medication to use for a particular patient. In preschool children, medication should only be considered for those individuals who have shown minimal benefit with PTBM and have significant behaviors interfering with daily functioning (Chang et. al, 2020). Medication management will be further discussed in chapter 7.

ADHD affects school performance. Supportive services at school may be necessary to ensure academic achievement. Many students with ADHD are eligible for accommodations and additional learning services. When minimal modifications are needed to optimize learning, a 504 plan may be recommended. When learning is significantly impaired by ADHD, school-based support such as occupational therapy may be included in a more inclusive individualized education program (IEP). 504s and IEPs are discussed in further detail in chapter 3.

D: Disruptive Behaviors

Thus far, I have described anxiety related disorders, mood disorders, and attention deficit/hyperactivity disorders. As a parent of children struggling with mental health, I agree these diagnoses may seem "disruptive" to the home and school environment. When I discuss disruptive behaviors, however, I am referring to an ongoing pattern of uncooperating and defiant action. Youngsters with this condition may respond to authority figures ranging from indifference to hostility. Their conduct impacts those around them including family, peers, and teachers. The most common types of disruptive behavior disorder are Oppositional Defiant Disorder (ODD) and Conduct Disorder (CD).

Oppositional Defiant Disorder

ODD is characterized by a pattern of angry or irritable mood, argumentative or defiant behavior, or vindictiveness lasting for at least six months (Riley et. al, 2016). Children may struggle to control their temper and are often disobedient. Typically, ODD manifests by late preschool or early elementary school age, though it can emerge in adolescence (Riley et. al, 2016). Parental concerns regarding ODD are a common reason patients present to my office for mental health services.

Like other conditions reviewed, the etiology of ODD is not well defined. Many experts believe the cause is multifactorial involving risk factors that stem from biological, psychological, and social issues. ODD is more frequent in children who live in poverty (Riley et. al, 2016). It generally affects boys more frequently than girls before adolescents, though this difference resolves in adolescence. Newer studies suggest parental behavior is more likely a cause rather than a response to the child's symptoms (Riley et. al, 2016). Social support is, therefore, a protective factor.

Janel was excited to get her learner's permit when she turned 15 years old. Her parents were a little nervous about teaching her to drive. Janel liked to do things her own way. She did not want anyone to show her how to do things. She preferred to learn from her own mistakes. Her parents were worried if they got in the passenger side of the car, and placed Janel in the driver's seat, it would only be a matter of time before she lost her temper with their instructions. Janel and her parents sat down and had a long conversation about her driving privileges.

"Now, you understand that driving a vehicle is a very serious endeavor," her father started out.

"I get it," Janel responded. "You have a lot of experience, and I am learning how to use the car. I promise I will listen to you and mom and only do what you tell me." It seemed too easy to get Janel to understand what she was taking on, yet her parents knew at some point they would need to teach her the skill of driving.

"If you argue with either of our instructions, the lesson is over and we are going home," her father continued.

"I know!" Janel returned.

Janel and her father went to an empty parking lot to start the first lesson. Her father tried to teach her the basic skills of getting the driver's seat in the right location, fixing the side and rearview mirrors, and how to navigate the various workings of the vehicle. "I learned all of this in the online driving class. Can't we just go?" Janel questioned.

"Remember, if we cannot get through the basics of how the car works and be sure you are sitting in an appropriate position to visibly see all areas outside the car, we are not going to continue with driving today and we are going to go home." Her father was already worried *about taking this lesson any further, but he hoped he could keep his patience going a little longer.*

Janel replied with her typical, "Fine."

After another ten minutes of education, Janel's father had her turn on the car, and she slowly made her way through the parking lot. They drove around for a bit while Janel got used to the maneuvers of the car. Her confidence rose quickly, faster than her father thought it should be. "Slow it down Janel," he requested.

"It's fine," Janel snapped. "I can do this."

Janel hit the accelerator of the car going through the turns of the lot a little faster to show her father she was competent. "Janel, I said slow down!" Her father raised his voice.

"I'm okay!" she shouted at him.

"Stop the vehicle," her father told her. "If you cannot listen, we are not doing this anymore today." Janel slammed on the break at once.

"Ugh!" Janel groaned. "You never let me do anything. I hate driving with you."

Individuals with ODD demonstrate a pattern of irritability, defiance, and vindictiveness more days than not (American Psychiatric Association, 2013). Because many oppositional behaviors are a normal part of early childhood into adolescence, the DSM-V now provides guidance of when these behaviors deviate from normal development. For example, throwing a temper tantrum in elementary school may be normal, but when it is a significant impairment such that the child is asked to leave school, it is not.

The DSM-V requirement to qualify an individual for a diagnosis of ODD includes patterns of irritable mood, argumentative behavior, or vindictiveness (American Psychiatric Association, 2013). Angry mood may be demonstrated by losing their temper frequently, becoming annoyed easily, or demonstrating resentfulness often. Defiant behaviors are noted when the individual often argues with authority figures, refuses to comply with requests or follow the rules, deliberately annoys others, or regularly blames others for mistakes the individual made. Individuals who are vindictive are spiteful and disposed to seek revenge (American Psychiatric Association, 2013). The DSM-V notes an individual with ODD must demonstrate a number of these behaviors for at least six months and their behavior leads to distress in their environment. To be declared ODD, the disturbance cannot be attributed to a medical condition, substance (such as a medication), or another mental health disorder (American Psychiatric Association, 2013). The severity of ODD is determined by the number of symptoms observed in the individual and the number of settings affected by the individual (American Psychiatric Association, 2013).

There are not any questionnaires specifically designed to screen for ODD. There are some tools that can aid in diagnosis while assessing other mental health conditions. In my practice, I most commonly use the National Institute for Children's Health Quality Vanderbilt Assessment Scale. This is a free questionnaire that is given to both parents and teachers to assess a child's behavior. The questionnaires are then returned to my office for review and a telephone or video visit is set up to discuss the findings with the child's parents. Other screening tools for evaluating ODD include Child Behavior Checklist, Swanson, Nolan and Pelham Teacher and Parent Rating Scale, and Conners Third Edition (Riley et. al, 2016).

ODD is generally not listed as a sole mental health ailment. Many children have additional mental health diagnoses. The most common comorbid condition seen with ODD is ADHD. Estimates of up to 40% of children with ODD have also been also identified with having ADHD (Riley et. al, 2016). While older studies suggested CD to be a more severe, age-related progression of ODD, it is now thought ODD and CD are separate conditions. Retrospective studies report CD is co-existent in up to 42% of individuals with ODD (Riley et. al, 2016). Anxiety and depression are commonly associated with ODD and can develop as early as preschool age. One report indicated 14% of children with ODD had anxiety and as many as 9% had a depressive disorder (Riley et. al, 2016). Those with angry symptoms of ODD are more likely to have mood disorders, whereas those with defiant and vindictive tendences are at a higher risk for CD. Substance use and other behavioral problems are also frequently seen in adolescents with ODD (Riley et. al, 2016).

Conduct Disorder

CD is characterized by repetitive, persistent violations of both the rights of others as well as age-appropriate social norms (Lillig, 2018). The average estimated lifetime prevalence of CD in the United States is 9%. CD is more commonly seen in males (12%) than it is in females (7.1%) (Lillig, 2018). Individuals may fit in one of many categories to be considered to have CD including aggression towards people or animals, property destruction, theft or deceitfulness, and serious rule violations (Lillig, 2018).

The etiology for CD may come from physiological, psychological, or social means. Risk factors for developing CD are increased in those with a maternal smoking history during pregnancy, individuals living in poverty, and parental conditions where substance use or criminal behaviors took place (Lillig, 2018). Additional risks for CD include exposure to physical or sexual abuse during childhood, witnessing domestic violence between parents, family instability, and associating with peers who utilize substances, skip school, or engage in illegal activities (Lillig, 2018)

Lucas is a 13 year old who came to my office with his mother for a well child checkup. "How are things going?" I asked Lucas and his mother.

"I don't know how I'm going to make it another five years with him!" Lucas' mother replied. "He sneaks out at night. He was caught vaping in the bathroom at school. His grades are poor, and he has no desire to change them. He was suspended for bullying a boy at school. I even found a Nintendo Switch in his room I think he stole from another kid. His dad is incarcerated, and I think Lucas is going down the same path."

CD includes a repetitive pattern of behavior where major rules are frequently violated. The DSM-V provides for one overarching diagnosis of CD but is specified by whether CD was childhood-onset type, adolescent-onset type, or unspecified onset (American Psychiatric Association, 2013). The DSM-V explains an individual may qualify for a diagnosis of CD if they have shown a repetitive pattern of behavior in which the basic rights of others are violated. Symptoms of CD are broken down into four categories: aggression to people and animals, destruction of property, deceitfulness and theft, and serious violations of rules (American Psychiatric Association, 2013). Several criteria must be observed over a period of twelve months. The behavioral disturbance of an individual with CD is significant enough to impair functioning in their community and at home (American Psychiatric Association, 2013).

CD is classified by whether an individual shows limited prosocial emotions, lack of remorse, inability to provide empathy, is unconcerned about performance, or does not show emotion (Lillig, 2018). The severity of CD may be categorized as mild, moderate, or severe. To be declared CD, the disturbance cannot be attributed to a medical condition, substance (such as a medication), or another mental health disorder. If the individual is over the age of 18, criteria for antisocial personality disorder will not qualify them for CD (American Psychiatric Association, 2013).

Like ODD, there are not any questionnaires specifically designed to screen for CD. There are some tools that can aid in diagnosis while assessing other mental health conditions. In my practice, I most commonly use the National Institute for Children's Health Quality Vanderbilt Assessment Scale. This is a free questionnaire that is given to both parents and teachers to assess a child's behavior. The questionnaires are then returned to my office for review and a telephone or video visit is set up to discuss the findings with the child's parents. Other screening tools include the Child Behavior Checklist and the Disruptive Behavior Disorders Rating Scale (Lillig, 2018).

The differential diagnosis for CD includes screening for other mental health ailments in which disruptive or aggressive actions may be present. To properly diagnose CD, conditions such as ODD, ADHD, mood disorders, adjustment disorders, and substance abuse must also be evaluated. There is a strong association of CD with ODD, ADHD, and substance use disorders (Lillig, 2018). In youth, the combined diagnosis of CD and ADHD may indicate a strong correlation to later tobacco and alcohol use. Adolescents with CD are less likely to complete high school and more likely to serve time in prison (Lillig, 2018). To help a youngster diagnosed with CD, treatment must support the family unit, psychosocial development, and in some cases include pharmacotherapy.

E: Eating Disorders

Ashley is 17 years old. Recently she set two school records for her high school swim team. She gets up regularly at 4:00 a.m. to be at school by 5:00 a.m. She swims for at least an hour before school and works out in the school's gym after classes are done for the day. Ashley skips breakfast because she "doesn't have time between morning swim and first period." She eats a salad for lunch and maybe a granola bar for dinner. Ashley is tall and very thin. She did not start her menstrual cycle until she was almost 16 years old and over the past year her periods have been very infrequent. When her mother tells her "You look pale, are you feeling okay?" Ashley just groans and walks away.

Jacob is 15 years old. At his last well child visit with his pediatrician his blood pressure and weight had increased significantly over the past year. His physician ordered some blood work that showed Jacob had pre-diabetes and elevated cholesterol. When his doctor asked him about his daily diet his responses were vague. That weekend, Jacob's mother decided his bedroom was overdue for a deep clean. She started working with Jacob to clean out his dressers and closet. Upon opening Jacob's closet, she saw several food wrappers thrown about.

"Jacob, I'm concerned about the amount of trash, specifically related to food, you have in your closet. What's going on?" his mother asked.

Shamefully, Jacob looked at the ground and shrugged his shoulders. "I just feel better when I'm sad and then I eat something," he replied.

Lauren is six years old. She started first grade. Her teacher has noticed that when Lauren is outdoors for recess, she spends a lot of time playing in the dirt. Most recently, her teacher has seen her eating the dirt. When her teacher tells her to stop, Lauren replies, "Why? I do it at home too."

Eating disorders are potentially life-threatening conditions characterized by disordered eating that impairs physical health and psychosocial functioning (Klein et. al, 2021). Adolescence and early adulthood are vulnerable times for developing eating disorders. Up to 8% of females and 2% of males will suffer from an abnormal eating condition during their lifetime (Klein et. al, 2021). Eating disorders affect individuals of all ages, sizes, sexual and gender groups, races, ethnicities, socioeconomic status, and geographical locations. Eating disorders often co-occur with mood, anxiety, substance use, personality, and somatic disorders. Even after treatment, many individuals with disordered eating have persistent symptoms that remain 20 years postdiagnosis (Klein et. al, 2021).

An individual's motivation to change may be compromised by malnutrition or co-occurring conditions, lack of self-awareness, or fear (Klein et. al, 2021). Individuals may use disordered eating to find perceived structure and safety in coping with difficult stressors (Klein et. al, 2021). Eating disorders are very challenging to treat. An individual is likely to have several members involved in their care team such as psychiatry, psychology, dietary, family counseling, and group therapy. There are various forms of eating disorders: anorexia nervosa, bulimia nervosa, binge-eating disorder, avoidant/restrictive food intake disorder, rumination disorder, and pica.

Common Eating Disorders (Klein et. al, 2021)

Anorexia Nervosa –

Individuals display with an intense fear of gaining weight. They have a distorted body image and restrict their intake of food to maintain a significantly low body weight. Atypical anorexia nervosa may be diagnosed when an individual restricts caloric intake, but their weight is not significantly affected.

Bulimia Nervosa –

Individuals place a great deal of their self-worth on their body shape and weight. When facing a perceived loss of control, they are likely to overindulge in caloric intake and then attempt to rid the calories in unhealthy ways to prevent weight gain. These individuals frequently misuse laxatives and diuretics. They may use vomiting, food restriction, or excessive exercise to avoid increased weight. Behaviors must occur at least weekly for at least three months and are distinctly separate from anorexia nervosa.

Binge-Eating Disorder –

Individuals are likely to overindulge in caloric intake when faced with perceived loss of control. These individuals are different than bulimia nervosa in that they do not have behaviors to prevent weight gain. Binge-eating disorder can be diagnosed when an individual has at least three of the following: eating faster than normal, eating until feeling uncomfortable, eating large quantities of food when not hungry, feeling bad because of embarrassment about eating behaviors, or eating followed by negative emotions. Behaviors must occur at least weekly for at least three months and are distinctly separate from anorexia nervosa or bulimia nervosa.

Avoidant/Restrictive Food Intake Disorder –

Individuals avoid food intake because of one of the following: lack of interest, sensory characteristics of food, or concern about consequences of eating that lead to unmet nutritional or energy needs. The individual is unaffected by body weight or shape. The eating pattern is not explained by food availability, culturally sanctioned practice, or specific medical or mental health condition. The individual is likely to suffer significant weight loss, inadequate weight gain during growth, nutritional deficiency, interference with psychosocial functioning, or dependence on supplemental feeding.

Rumination Disorder –

Individuals have repeated regurgitation of food for at least one month, not attributable to a medical condition, and not occurring secondary to another eating disorder.

Pica –

Individuals are known to engage in eating nonnutritive, nonfood substances for at least one month, eating behavior is developmentally inappropriate, and not part of culturally supported practices.

Restoring an individual's healthy relationship with food involves fostering cognitive flexibility around eating, removal of harmful behaviors, and reducing body dissatisfaction (Klein et. al, 2021). Addressing disordered eating early on helps decrease the risk of long-term pathology. Medication management should not be used as a single treatment option. A full care team is needed for effective treatment. For youths with an eating disorder, family therapy is very important in treatment success.

F: Gender Dysphoria

A 12-year-old patient and her mother visited my clinic with a request for menstrual cycle suppression. Assigned at birth as female, my patient identified as male from a very early age. He primarily had male friends, dressed in clothes from the boy's department, and played only on co-ed sports teams. When he developed breast buds, he started showing signs of depressed mood. He started wearing larger clothes to hide the physical changes. His mother was very supportive of her child and was able to find breast binding materials to conceal breast tissue. Two years later, he started having menstrual cycles. My patient became very distraught. He had both increased anxiety and depression. To suppress menstrual cycles, I started oral contraception, however, when this did not work the first month, and he had another period, he took most of the hormone pack of pills to try and stop the bleeding.

Determining one's sex is straightforward. Generally, there is a second trimester ultrasound image, which is later consistent with external genitalia at birth, and biological sex of male or female is recorded on the birth certificate. In contrast to biological sex, gender identity is an individual's inner knowledge of who they are: man, woman, or something else (Turban, 2020). Gender identity is not understood as clearly as biological sex. In the United States, gender has historically been defined as man or woman. Some cultures, however, have long recognized gender identities outside of this binary. "Fa'afafine" in Samoan society, "two spirit" in indigenous North American culture, and "hijra" in South Asia are three examples (Fabiani, 2021). Gender identity develops as early as two years of age and children have a consistent understanding of their own gender identity by age four (Rafferty, 2022).

In the United States, approximately 150,000 youth and 1.4 million adults identify as transgender (Klein et. al, 2018). Transgender describes individuals who expressed gender differs from their sex assigned at birth. Gender dysphoria occurs when this gender incongruence causes significant distress (Klein et. al, 2018). Gender dysphoria, previously termed gender identity disorder, is a term that should be used to describe distressing symptoms rather than to pathologize (Klein et. al, 2018). In transgender individuals, sexual orientation, sex development, or external gender expression should not be assumed. It is equally important not to assume the individual's sexual or romantic attraction based on their asserted gender.

Transgender individuals are known to have high rates of mental health diagnoses (Klein et. al, 2018). A person's mental health condition, however, may not be related to being transgender and other causes should be evaluated. For many sexual-minority youth, they are often challenged by suicidality, body image distortion, substance abuse, and high-risk sexual behavior (Klein et. al, 2018). Often these ailments stem from the effects of an unsupportive environment. In adolescents meeting the diagnostic criteria for gender dysphoria, suppression of pubertal hormones may be indicated while the individual worked with a trained clinician to affirm their sense of self and explore their gender identity further. Puberty-blocking and gender-affirming hormone treatment is not generally recommended in prepubertal children (Wilkes, 2018). When indicated, gonadotropin-releasing hormone analogues may be used to delay further pubertal changes. Sex hormone therapy, including estrogen and testosterone (which may have partially irreversible effects), should be initiated using a gradual dose schedule only after a team of medical and mental health professionals confirm the persistence of gender dysphoria and mental capacity of informed consent (Wilkes, 2018).

There is no universally accepted treatment protocol for prepubertal gender-diverse children (Klein et. al, 2018). Transgender adolescents should have access to psychological therapy for support and a safe means to explore their gender identity. Once an individual reaches late puberty or adulthood, cross-sex hormone therapy appears to improve mental health outcomes and quality of life for transgender persons (Klein et. al, 2018). Surgical options may further decrease gender dysphoria and may decrease required doses of hormones. Unfortunately, surgeries are not always covered by health insurance making them cost-prohibitive for many individuals (Klein et. al, 2018).

The DSM-V provides for one overarching diagnosis of gender dysphoria, but with separate specific criteria for children and for adolescents and adults. The DSM-V stipulates children may qualify for a diagnosis of gender dysphoria disorder if they have a strong desire to be an alternative gender to their assigned gender, desire to wear clothing of their expressed gender, preference for cross-gender roles in fantasy play, a strong dislike of their sexual anatomy, and longing for physical sex characteristics that match their preferred gender (American Psychiatric Association, 2013). The condition must last at least six months and interfere with optimal functioning at home or school. For adolescents, the DSM-V goes into additional detail describing a strong feeling to rid the individual's own secondary sex characteristics, be treated as the other gender, and a personal conviction to respond to situations as their expressed gender (American Psychiatric Association, 2013).

Putting It All Together

This chapter described the most common mental health ailments youngsters face. Diagnosing an adolescent may at first glance seem straightforward. For instance, complete an assessment tool to help guide the evaluation. Next, score the examination using the provided key and determine whether the child fits the benchmarks to be diagnosed with a condition. If the child tests positive for a diagnosis, schedule the appropriate treatment and medication appointments. Unfortunately, when it comes to kids, it is not so black and white. Adolescents are individuals with their own experiences, and they do not always follow a checklist of psychological traits.

Julia's Story

A pediatrician colleague of mine, Meera, shared her story about her youngest child, Julia. When Julia was in third grade, she woke up with a stomach-ache. Meera would immediately go into doctor mode. "Where does it hurt?"

"All over," Julia would say.

"Can you point to it with one finger?" Meera would ask.

Julia would rub her hands all over her abdomen in a circular motion making sure not to miss any areas.

"When did it start?"

"It hurt when I woke up."

"What makes it better?" Meera was in full pediatrician mode now.

"Nothing," Julia replied.

"What makes it worse?"

"I don't know," Julia mumbled. Meera should not have been surprised by her child's short, unhelpful answers, but these were the questions drilled into my colleague's head since she was a medical student. This was her default. Yet it was very frustrating on a Monday morning when she was trying to determine whether to send her child to school that day and her daughter was being, what we call in our world, a poor historian.

Meera felt Julia's forehead. Julia did not feel feverish. Meera examined her daughter's abdomen. It was soft, nondistended, and there was no specific tenderness when palpating the various quadrants. My colleague was at a loss.

"Are you hungry?"

"No," Julia said.

"Do you feel like you're going to throw up? Do you feel like you need to use the bathroom?"

"I don't think so."

The child looked as though she did not feel good. Julia appeared as though she needed to rest. "I'll call into work and spend the day here with you," Meera told her.

One day of an upset stomach for a school aged kid is common. It seemed like a viral bug. Elementary kids can be a large petri dish of germs. My colleague was certain her daughter picked up something from a classmate.

The illnesses became frequent. First it was a stomach-ache, then headaches. Sometimes Julia would feel ill for two or three days at a time. Meera took her child to the pediatrician's office. Sometimes providing healthcare to family is detrimental. Doctors can be too close to a loved one and misread a situation leading to a false idea of how to be able to treat the symptoms. My colleague was worried she was too close to her child to see what was causing Julia's discomfort. The pediatrician, however, was also unsure why Julia had so many physical concerns.

During this time, Julia's father and mother were not doing well in their marriage. They tried to avoid fighting in front of the kids, but they were clearly unhappy. A few times Julia walked in on her mother crying in the corner of her bedroom wishing things were different.

"What's wrong?" Julia would say as she gave her mother a hug.

"Sometimes grown-ups are just sad," Meera would tell her as she wiped her eyes and stood up to help Julia with whatever led her daughter to search for Meera in the first place.

Julia did not experience sadness in the way my colleague was feeling those same emotions at the end of a dysfunctional marriage. My colleague showed signs of fatigue and tearfulness. She overslept. She searched for food to fill the void she felt. Julia had only stomach pain and headaches. My colleague understood the basis of her depression. Julia only felt physical pain and did not understand its origin. Diagnosing a mental health condition in a child can be a challenging task. A child may demonstrate anxiety through physical aggression instead of restlessness. A cry for help may come as defiance and acting out. Screening tools may help providers identify where to start treatment but finding the source of a child's emotions may take many therapeutic sessions.

A diagnosis in an adolescent may not be concrete. In my experience, providers are not quick to label a child with a particular ailment such as "bipolar" or "conduct disorder." The mind of a child is fluid and changes based on their experiences. When I have a teenager in my office talking over their parent with a "know it all" tone I educate them on the fact they do not have an adult brain until they are at least in their mid-twenties (Arain, 2013). The limbic system is the part of the brain that helps a developing adolescent take in their environment, determine a response to stimuli, and store it for later use (Smith, 2015). Youngsters' brains process information in a fascinating way. Their brains are constantly taking in new data and their personality may transform over time, making a diagnosis made during a time of life stressors no longer appropriate. "Why diagnose them at all?" you may wonder. Diagnosis helps lead treatment. It tells the care team "this is where to start." In other words, a diagnosis supports a path for therapeutic intervention.

You may have noticed I did not cover personality disorders in this chapter. With an adolescent brain being so malleable, it's often hard to determine whether a characteristic is a true personality trait, or a phase of development. In my professional experience, during adolescence a diagnosis may need to be re-visited every couple of years to see if the current course of treatment is still appropriate or if another pathway would be more fitting.

*Homework: Your Child's Diagnosis (Additional Matter –
Your Child's Characteristics).*

Chapter 6

ALPHABET SOUP OF THERAPY

ddie closed her eyes. She felt the warmth of the black leather chaise surround her body as she lay stretched across it. Her head was cradled by a large fluffy pillow. Sitting behind the head of the couch, her therapist sat in an upright chair covered in red fabric. The therapist had her brown hair tied neatly in a bun behind her head. Through her glasses, the therapist looked onto a long legal pad, supported by her crossed legs. A fountain pen was in her right hand, ready to take notes of the session. "How does that make you feel Addie?" the therapist questioned.

When many individuals think of therapy, they visualize lying on a lounger while a professional asks them how they feel about a particular situation. This idea of therapy is best assigned to Sigmund Freud, an Austrian neurologist, and the founder of psychoanalysis. Freud used this cough/chair set up to change the pace of typical social interactions (Kunst, 2014). When individuals interact face-to-face, they are held by eye contact and facial expressions. While there is a place for this type of social connection, there is an implicit pressure to be polite, smile, and show understanding (Kunst, 2014). In contrast, looking away from the therapist and lying comfortably may allow an individual comfort to think more freely. The individual is permitted to escape expectations of conversational interactions. They may find value in letting their thoughts wander, gaining access to their unconscious mind (Kunst, 2014).

Psychoanalysis is not the only form of therapy. In my experience as a medical professional, asking a child or adolescent to first lie on a couch, trust me, and tell me their deepest feelings is likely to be met with resistance. In my experience as a parent, I would expect this situation to result in my child getting up and walking out of the room after making some sarcastic remark. When my children first started needing a therapeutic approach to help with mental distress, I was amazed at the number of approaches to therapy that were available. Just as no two individuals are alike, therapeutic approach is not a "one size fits all."

When I first went into medicine, it was not uncommon for a primary care physician to divide their time taking care of patients in the hospital in the morning and in the office setting in the afternoon. With the advancement of information technology, sharing of medical knowledge increased. Evidence-based medicine became popularized. It was challenging for providers to "specialize" in both hospital-based medicine and office-based medicine. Two types of primary care providers emerged, those that treated patients when they were in the hospital (hospitalists) and those that treated patients when they were not in the hospital (ambulatory). Behavioral health has gone a similar way. There are many therapists available who specialize in different therapeutic approaches. In our current healthcare setting, it is not uncommon for a patient to have more than one mental health provider.

When you are new to therapy, the acronyms can feel overwhelming. CBT. DBT. EMDR. PBMT. AAT. The list goes on. What are all these approaches? How do you know what method is best for your child? When do you need to include more than one method? Fortunately, as the parent, you are not required to make this decision. If you've involved a good behavioral health provider, they will spend time getting to know your child and determining the best treatment plan for the situation. I have found it advantageous as a parent to understand the type of help my child is receiving.

Therapeutic Lifestyle Changes (TLC)

Therapeutic lifestyle changes are activities of daily living which can be incorporated in the home to provide improvement in mental wellbeing. While a trained professional may suggest certain techniques, they are only with your child for one hour every week or two. Parents can take the lead by helping integrate these skills into the household. Since children are very observant, the best way you can influence your child is by modeling the behaviors you wish to see. If you establish that physical activity, for example, is important, yet your children never see you exercise, they may not feel inclined to increase exercise. Similarly, if the therapist recommends emotional regulation skills, such as deep breathing, you should follow up with your child to see they are practicing these techniques between counseling sessions. Types of therapeutic lifestyle changes include:

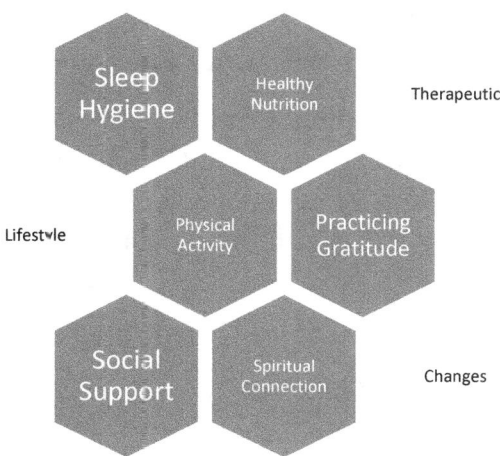

Sleep is a cornerstone to mental health. Sleep allows the brain and the body to heal. When children do not get enough sleep, they may become irritable, lack focus, and exhibit anxiety. School aged children require between nine and 12 hours of sleep each night, yet many only receive seven to eight hours. Teenagers require eight to ten hours of sleep per 24 hours (CDC, 2020). The American Sleep Association defines sleep hygiene as behaviors that one can do to help promote quality sleep (American Sleep Association, 2022). Sleep hygiene tips include:

1. Maintain a regular sleep routine. Go to bed at the same time every day. Wake up at the same time every day.

2. Avoid daytime naps. When an individual sleeps during the day, it reduces the amount of overall sleep that is needed. This may cause difficulty falling asleep at night and sleep fragmentation.

3. Do not stay awake in bed for more than five to ten minutes. The bed should be for sleep only. The body will come to recognize the bed as a place for rest. If the mind is racing, the individual should get up, sit in a chair in the dark for a few minutes until the brain is tired, and then return to bed again. Focusing on electronics such as TV, social media, and the internet use during these periods will restimulate the brain and should be avoided.

4. Avoid electronic stimuli for 30 minutes before going to bed. Never watch TV or use the phone or computer in bed. Blue light from screen activity can adversely affect the circadian rhythm. Using an inexpensive pair of blue light blocking glasses or using a blue light filter two hours before bed has been shown to improve duration and quality of sleep.

5. The effects of caffeine may last several hours after ingestion. Caffeine may cause difficulty with sleep initiation and fragment sleep. Caffeine use should be used prior to noon.

6. Other substances that interfere with sleep include cigarettes, alcohol, and many over the counter medications, such as cold medicines.

7. Cracking a window allows for plenty of fresh air to help with sleep quality.

8. Exercise promotes quality sleep but should be done before two in the afternoon. Rigorous physical activity circulates endorphins within the body which may make sleep initiation more challenging.

9. Have a quiet, comfortable bedroom. The bedroom should be a dark place without distractions. If the bedroom is too hot or too cold, it may be difficult to maintain sleep. If a pet awakens an individual, they may not be a helpful accommodation for rest.

10. Have a calm bedtime routine such as taking a warm bath or shower or meditating.

A healthy diet supports mental wellbeing. What we eat affects our energy levels and affects our mood. When sugar is absorbed, it acts on the brain to disrupt normal neurochemical physiology (Greenblatt & Ross-Taylor, 2019). Typically, after a large meal, a hormone known as ghrelin is suppressed telling the brain it is no longer hungry. Sugar interferes with the suppression of ghrelin. Sugar blocks the transport of the hormone leptin. Release of leptin leads to the feeling of fullness; without it an individual remains hungry (Greenblatt & Ross-Taylor, 2019). Sugar weakens dopamine signaling in the brain's reward center. Dopamine is the pleasure hormone. Sugar increases dopamine release so individuals feel more pleasure after its consumption (Greenblatt & Ross-Taylor, 2019).

Researchers have studied animal behavior and neurochemistry to better understand the biological basis of food addiction. When researchers gave rats a sugar solution, the solution increased the release of the pleasure hormone, dopamine, in their brain (Greenblatt & Ross-Taylor, 2019). Over time, the rat's brain stopped producing its own natural dopamine and the rats required more and more of the substance to get a pleasurable effect. When the sugar solution was withdrawn from the rats, the rats demonstrated signs of anxiety and physical dependence. The rats were too anxious to explore their surroundings and remained huddled in a tunnel, teeth chattering, and startling easily (Greenblatt & Ross-Taylor, 2019).

Interestingly, additional studies have demonstrated similar changes in the brain from sugar addiction as seen in alcohol dependence. While a parent would not consider giving their child whiskey for breakfast, pack a wine cooler for lunch, and serve a beer with dinner, how often do we present our child with orange juice and pancakes for breakfast, peanut butter and jelly sandwich with pretzels and fruit snacks for lunch, then pizza for dinner? The Standard American Diet tends to lean towards processed foods, on-the-go foods, and sugar/carbohydrate dense foods. Introducing your child to a nutritionally sound meal plan with a combination of protein, vegetables, fruit, and complex carbohydrates can significantly improve their mood. My daughter found working with a nutrition specialist was just as critical to her mental health as meeting with her counselor.

The benefits of exercise on physical and mental health are well documented. Exercise improves mental health by reducing negative moods that may trigger anxiety and depression. Exercise has been demonstrated to improve self-esteem and cognitive function (Charles, 2022). If a child is burdened by illness, pain, or hopelessness they may see several barriers to physical activity. Talk openly with your child about their concerns. Actively listen to your child so they feel as though they are being heard. For example, if your child says "I'm bad at sports. I can't exercise because it will make me feel worse about myself," perhaps you can respond with, "I hear you feel you are not very good at playing sports. Perhaps you have never found an activity that was right for you. What if we find one we can do together?" Set realistic and attainable activity goals with your child. Initially finding things you can do alongside your child may keep them engaged.

I love the outdoors. I enjoy listening to the birds and watching nature while drinking my morning coffee on the back porch during the summer. I crave sunshine. The fact I have chosen residence in a state that is partly cloudy year-round astounds me. Light therapy is a way to treat seasonal affective disorder and certain other conditions by exposure to artificial light when true sunlight is lacking. Bright white light exposure within the first hour of waking and for approximately 20 to 30 minutes can be effective in improving mood in some individuals (Mayo Clinic, 2022). You can purchase light therapy devices for less than 30 dollars.

When possible, getting outdoors reduces symptoms of anxiety and depression. An analysis of 10 studies found that spending time in a green environment improved both mood and self-esteem (Lifeworks, 2020). Earthing, also known as grounding, refers to contact with the Earth's surface electrons by walking barefoot outside. This practice allows transfer of energy from the ground into the body, stabilizing the body's physiology at the deepest levels and promoting great wellbeing. Environmental medicine research shows promising results on mental and physical health when individuals are reconnected to nature (Chevalier et. al, 2012).

Gratitude is the quality of being thankful. An individual who is demonstrating gratitude is ready to show appreciation and kindness. Gratitude is focusing on the positive things in life, no matter how big or how small the event may be. Gratitude journals have become popular in the last few years. There are many options for purchasing a gratitude journal. A simple notebook is also an acceptable tool for accomplishing this therapeutic modality. Writing down blessings you have experienced, even once a week, has been shown to boost mood. When I have actively maintained a gratitude journal, I have found myself looking for positive experiences in my daily life to be able to document within its pages.

Human beings are a social species. Neither society nor the individual exists in isolation. Each is dependent on one another. Social interaction is essential to every aspect of our health. Having a strong network of support fosters an individual both emotionally and physically. When I screen for mental wellbeing in the office, I include social determinants of health. I want to know how often my patients talk to friends or family, get together with others to spend time in person. I am curious about whether my patient belongs to any clubs or organizations and how often they meet with other members. How an individual identifies within the family unit is also crucial for emotional security.

As discussed in chapter two, spirituality has a profound effect on mental health. Spirituality and religion are not necessarily congruent. A spiritual individual is one that can connect with their surroundings. In my experience, people who bond with the world around them are more likely to find inner peace. Knowing one's place as it relates to a bigger whole can bring about a sense of purpose. One way to be present in the moment is by learning how to meditate. Children and adolescents may find meditation initially challenging. Today's youngster is surrounded by the ever-changing, ever-stimulating online world. Images and thoughts in the tech world sometimes move faster than we can observe in the real world. Slowing down the brain to be present with the world we currently have access to may feel unnatural. That's fine! It is okay to feel uncomfortable at first. Over time, the unpleasant feelings will fade.

If you are new to meditation, I suggest the following:

Find somewhere you can relax. This should be a location that is quiet and without a lot of distractions. Take a seat. Start by setting a timer for five minutes. Close your eyes. Notice your body. Is there tension? Where? Does the tension go anywhere else? Do you have pain? Does the pain travel? Get to know your body's position and feel its response to gentle shifting. Feel your breath. Follow the sensation of your breath as it goes in and as it goes out. Notice your mind. Notice if your mind wanders. This is normal. When you find your mind drifting from the present, bring your thoughts back to your breath in the moment. Be kind to your wandering mind. Don't judge yourself over the content of the thoughts you find yourself lost in. Come back to the moment. Close with kindness. When you are ready to continue your day, gently open your eyes and notice any sounds in your environment. Notice your body. Notice your emotions. Be content with the you that is facing the day.

Poor mental health often involves a vicious cycle of sad mood, fatigue, social isolation, and avoidance of activity. This withdrawal can further exacerbate the declining emotional wellbeing. Behavioral activation is an approach to improved mental health that starts by having an individual understand the behaviors leading to their current state. Individuals are then encouraged to identify things they once found exciting. Through behavioral activation, treatment focuses on increasing engagement in the identified pleasant activities.

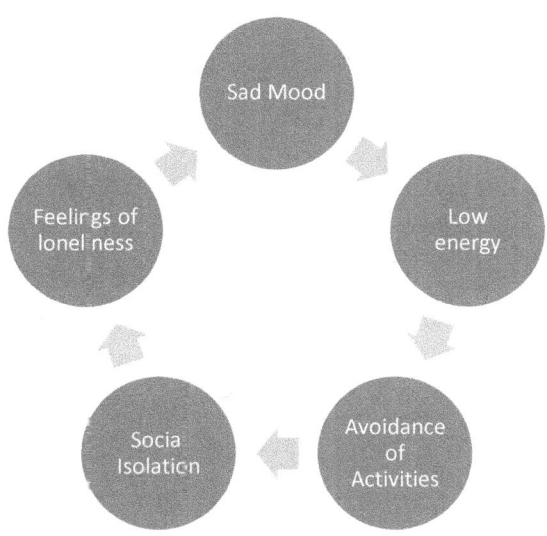

Cycle of Poor Mental Health

You can empower your child to break the cycle of mental anguish by explaining the cycle, noting the consequences of continued avoidance and isolation, and urging them to engage in some type of pleasurable activity, even if they do not yet feel like doing so. It may be helpful for your child to understand if you draw a picture of the cycle on paper and plan the behaviors in advance. Tracking moods before and after activities may also help yield persuasive data to encourage continued activity. If a child wants to wait to feel better before engaging in activities, that time may not come. Behavioral activation requires participation in an activity regardless of mood or energy level.

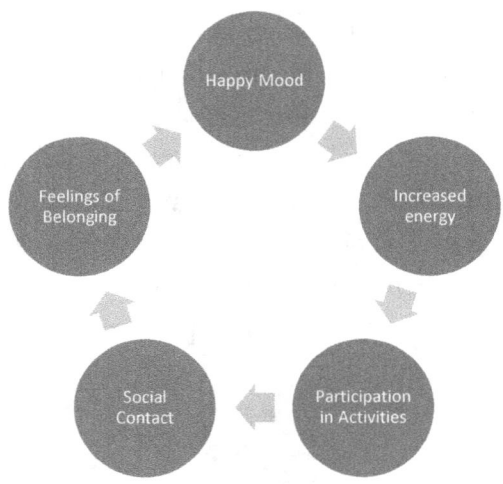

Cycle Leading to Good Mental Health

Individuals struggling with depression, anxiety, or other ailments may benefit from creating routines or schedules. Generating a routine provides structure. It invites the individual to get out of bed in the morning to complete a task. My patients often report their mood and overall quality of life improves when they are busier.

Anticipate that your adolescent will be hesitant about the helpfulness of this tool. This reaction is likely part of their negative state of thinking. You may hear your child say, "Nothing is fun," "My life is terrible," "No one wants to spend time with me." You may feel like you need to fix the situation and convince them things will improve. You cannot understand how they feel, and they know this. You can, however, respect their feelings and explore barriers with them to encourage a healthier approach. For example, "I hear that you are not finding anything fun to do right now. What did you find fun before? What made it no longer interesting? What would you do differently?""

Therapeutic lifestyle changes are things that can be encouraged within the household. A therapist may recommend a lifestyle change, but they do not spend as much time with your child as you do. Parents can be the biggest influences on how their children spend their day. The next therapeutic approaches are somewhat different. Specially trained professionals may opt to use one method over another to help your child work through their struggles. It's helpful to understand the tactic behind the approach, but as a parent, the best way to support your child is by checking in with their therapist regularly to see if there is anything you can do to help supplement the sessions at home.

Cognitive Behavioral Therapy (CBT)

Cognitive Behavioral Therapy (CBT) is a time limited, goal oriented, psychotherapy (Coffey et. al, 2015). CBT has been demonstrated to be effective for a range of ailments including anxiety and mood disorders, post-traumatic stress disorder, attention-deficit/hyperactivity disorder, autism spectrum disorder, obsessive-compulsive and tic disorders, substance abuse disorders, eating disorders, and many other severe mental illnesses (Coffey et. al, 2015). CBT is an approach that is supported by evidence-based research. In other words, CBT has been demonstrated to produce change. In this way, CBT differs from many other forms of psychological treatments.

CBT is based on three core principles. First, psychological difficulties are based on unhelpful ways of thinking (PTSD Clinical Practice Guideline, 2017). Miranda thinks, "I have no friends. No one wants to spend time with me." The continued irrational thinking leads to feelings of sadness, loneliness, or even anger at herself. The second concept of CBT considers mental health ailments are based, in part, on learned patterns of behavior (PTSD Clinical Practice Guideline, 2017). Returning to Miranda, emotions with an underlying tone of sorrow may lead to behaviors of isolation, overeating, or substance use. Further detachment from social support can lead Miranda to additional identification of being alone. The last concept of CBT is that individuals suffering with emotional disturbances can learn better ways of managing them, thereby reducing their symptoms, and becoming more effective in their lives (PTSD Clinical Practice Guideline, 2017). A counselor may challenge Miranda to change her behavior to promote improved ways of thinking and mending her feelings.

CBT encourages long term changes in behaviors and thought patterns. It is most effective when individuals complete therapeutic practices outside of the treatment session. A significant commitment from children and parents will improve successful treatment. A typical course of CBT is one 30-to-60-minute session once weekly, generally for five to 20 weeks (NHS, 2019). Symptoms are monitored frequently. Treatment is goal-oriented and collaborative. If a child does not desire to participate, CBT is less likely to be effective.

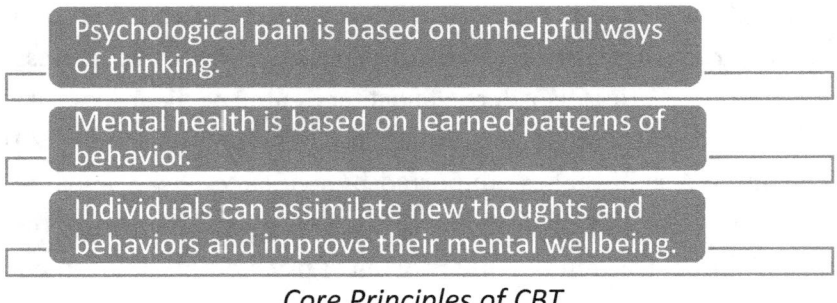

Core Principles of CBT

Cognitive Processing Therapy (CPT)

Cognitive Processing Therapy (CPT) is one specific type of cognitive behavioral therapy. CPT is a 12-session psychotherapy for individuals suffering from post-traumatic stress disorder (PTSD) (U.S. Department of Veterans Affairs, 2022). Each session is typically 60-90 minutes (Adikwu, 2020). CPT teaches individuals how to evaluate and change upsetting thoughts they may have after a significant trauma. Frequently, individuals with PTSD experience "stuck points." Stuck points are concise statements that reflect a thought. These points can keep the individual from recovering. The goal of CPT is to change one's thought pattern so that they may be able to improve the emotions and heal (Adikwu, 2020).

Eye Movement Desensitization and Reprocessing (EMDR)

Eye Movement Desensitization and Reprocessing (EMDR) is a psychotherapy treatment that was originally designed to alleviate distress associated with traumatic memories (EMDR Institute, 2020). Your child does not have to be a combat soldier to encounter trauma. The Centers for Disease Control and Prevention reports one in four girls and one in 13 boys in the United States experience sexual trauma. Many children wait to report or never report sexual abuse likely making that figure likely an underestimate of the true impact of the problem (CDC, 2021). Twelve percent of children 17 years of age and under live with at least one parent with an alcohol use disorder (NCDAS, 2022). While humans overall are a resilient species, traumatic experiences can leave their mark. Trauma not only affects the exposed individual, but also those who surround them.

Trauma is unbearable. It takes a great deal of energy to move from a life-shattering event to being productive and happy. At first, even day to day activities such as getting ready for school or work, meal preparation, and basic hygiene may seem overwhelming. To survive, trauma victims may try to compartmentalize. They may try to shove the experience into a sealed vault and tuck it away in the back of their brain to avoid thinking about the situation. While the victim wants to move on and believes thought avoidance to be beneficial in accomplishing that task, the part of the brain which ensures our survival is not very good at denial. Trauma produces actual physiological changes in the brain (Van der Kolk, 2014). Long after the disturbing event, the brain may be reactivated by the slightest hint of danger. Brain circuits will secrete stress hormones to cope with perceived danger (Van der Kolk, 2014). This may cause the individual to feel intense unpleasant physical sensations. Individuals may even respond impulsively and aggressively to combat their realized fear of the situation.

Severe emotional pain can require a great deal of time to recover. EMDR therapy helps the mind recover from psychological trauma, just as the body recovers from physical trauma (EMDR Institute, 2020). For instance, if you were working in the yard and a splinter wedged itself into your hand, you would feel significant physical pain. Removal of the foreign object would reduce the pain you felt. EMDR uses detailed protocols learned by providers in extensive training sessions to help patients activate their natural healing processes. Unlike talk therapy, the insight individuals gain after EMDR result more from their own accelerated emotional processing of the situation and less from clinical interpretation (EMDR Institute, 2020).

Most EMDR providers begin with a thorough history taking session. The therapist determines whether a client is ready to process their trauma and develops a treatment plan. It is important to identify specific skills the individual will need to acquire to be used in future situations. If it appears the individual is ready to begin processing their event, and EMDR treatment is appropriate, significant time is spent preparing them to be able to handle emotional distress. Your mental health provider should ensure your child has adequate resources available to handle increased stressors, should they be encountered, between therapy sessions. I have seen patients who have worked with EMDR specialists. The good outcomes have come from the providers that set up a safety plan prior to actual EMDR sessions. The safety plan included who to call if the patient was feeling anxious, what techniques to use to calm their emotions, and a crisis number in case the safety plan was ineffective.

The next phase of EMDR includes vivid imagery related to a specific memory, exploring negative thinking about oneself, and processing emotions and body sensations related to the event (EMDR Institute, 2020). The therapist helps the individual identify positive beliefs that can be used to replace unpleasant thoughts and feelings. The provider may introduce a technique of eye movement to help with emotional processing (Indiana Health Group, 2022). While facing the patient, the therapist will move their fingers to the right and to the left of their field of vision. The patient moves their eyes in step with the therapist's fingers. It is thought that this eye movement technique causes stimulation of both the right and left sides of the brain. This bilateral stimulation bypasses the area of the brain that became "stuck" due to the previous trauma. EMDR helps the left side of the brain self-soothe the right side of the brain while the clinician guides the patient through a process known as desensitization. Future sessions are devoted to reinforcing and strengthening positive beliefs until the patient gets to the point where the trauma can be discussed without experiencing the negativity that led to treatment in the first place (Indiana Health Group, 2022).

Dialectical Behavioral Therapy (DBT)

Dialectical Behavior Therapy (DBT) is a comprehensive, evidence-based treatment that began with efforts to treat personality disorders, specifically borderline personality disorder (Chapman, 2006). DBT is now being used to help individuals with mood disorders, suicidal ideation, and individuals who struggle with self-harming behaviors and substance abuse (Chapman, 2006). DBT is a type of talking therapy. While like CBT, it's been adapted for individuals who feel emotions very intensely. The goal of therapy is to help individuals understand and accept difficult feelings (Schimelpfening, 2021).

The standard DBT treatment package consists of weekly one-hour individual sessions, weekly two-hour group skills training sessions, and a therapist consultation team meeting. In this way, DBT is a comprehensive treatment program, rather than a single method conducted by a single provider. To be considered DBT, treatment must fulfill four functions. First, the patient has out of control behavior (Delray Center for Healing, 2022). They may be self-harming in various ways. The first goal is to move forward by gaining behavioral control. Second, while the harmful behavior may be eliminated, the patient continues to suffer in silence (Delray Center for Healing, 2022). The individual's emotional state is still inhibited. The goal of this stage is to help the patient move into an emotionally healthy space. Third, the patient needs to learn to live (Delray Center for Healing, 2022). Now that behaviors and emotions are in a healthy space, the individual must learn to live a functioning life. They must be able to handle the ups and downs that life brings. Lastly, patients learn to find a deeper meaning through a spiritual existence (Delray Center for Healing, 2022). Individuals work to gain a sense of connectedness from being part of a greater whole.

Mindfulness Based Stress Reduction (MBSR)

Mindfulness Based Stress Reduction (MBSR) is an eight-week evidence-based program that helps an individual learn strategies to reduce daily stress. Each session is between two and three hours in duration and focuses on one topic that is explored with exercises, a presentation from an instructor, and a dialogue among group participants (Institute for Mindfulness-Based Approaches, 2022). While initially targeted to people with chronic health problems, today MBSR is taught to people throughout the world who are experiencing challenges in all areas of life, medical and emotional. Through MBSR, people become familiar with their own behaviors, especially in response to stressful situations (Institute for Mindfulness-Based Approaches, 2022). The main exercises of MBSR include the body scan, gentle yoga, and sitting meditation. Participants are expected to practice one of these exercises daily. MBSR has been found to be useful in the treatment of chronic pain, anxiety, insomnia, fatigue, headaches, skin disorders and high blood pressure (Institute for Mindfulness-Based Approaches, 2022).

Mindfulness Based Cognitive Therapy (MBCT) is a method of helping people to stay well following successful CBT treatment. It combines the philosophy of CBT with MBSR to help prevent relapse.

Exposure Therapy

Exposure therapy was developed to help individuals face their fears (Clinical Practice Guideline for the Treatment of PTSD, 2017). When someone has an excessive fear of a particular object or situation, it can significantly interfere with their quality of life. Exposure therapy involves subjecting the individual to the source of the anxiety trigger slowly, and without the intent to cause any danger. By slowly introducing the person to the stimulus, they become desensitized over time and can overcome their fear.

For example, Logan is afraid of spiders. When he sees a spider in his room, he begins to experience significant distress. Last week, Logan saw a spider in the corner of his room near the ceiling. While the spider was small, Logan's heart began to race, and his stomach grew ill. Logan called his parents in panic to come into the room and get rid of the spider. If Logan were to participate in exposure therapy, the therapist might first talk to Logan about spiders. When Logan was able to have a conversation freely about a spider, Logan might move on to looking at pictures of spiders. Over time, Logan would hopefully find reviewing pictures of spiders to not be a trigger of his anxiousness. The process would continue to have Logan sit in a room with a spider in a cage, Logan sitting near the cage, Logan touching the cage, the lid of the cage being open, and eventually the goal would be that Logan could touch a spider without significant apprehension.

Solutions Focused Brief Therapy (SFBT)

Solutions Focused Brief Therapy (SFBT) is a future-focused, goal-directed treatment that focuses on solutions, rather than on the problems individuals are facing. SFBT is an evidence based therapeutic approach that incorporates positive psychology principles. It is a hope-friendly vehicle for formulating, motivating, achieving, and sustaining desired behavioral change (Institute for Solution-Focused Therapy, 2022).

SFBT begins with a detailed description of how the individual's life will be different when the situation has improved. The provider and the patient then work together to determine the resources the individual will need to produce a sustainable solution. Therapists and their patients continue to collaborate to identify the individual's goals and satisfying solutions.

Goals (Formulated from Individual's Desire for Change)

- What is the vision of the present? Future?
- What is the patient doing now to reach the goal?
- Is the goal appropriate for the patient's desired outcome?
- What are positive features of the patient's future once goals are obtained?

Solutions (Expectation Driven)

- What are specific steps needed to reach the goal?
- Describe an action plan measurable, realistic, and achievable.

When SFBT is ineffective, it is important to re-examine the individual's goals. What does the patient want? What has been left out of the solution plan? Do the goals need to be renegotiated? Was the therapy working in the wrong direction?

Acceptance and Commitment Therapy (ACT)

Acceptance and Commitment Therapy (ACT) is a form of psychotherapy that uses acceptance and mindfulness techniques, together with commitment and behavioral change strategies, to increase psychological flexibility (Ackerman, 2017). In other words:

| Acceptance & Mindfulness | + Commitment & Strageties to Modify Behavior | = Flexibility of the brain to deal with the environment in new ways |

As we have previously discussed, the brain has a way of perceiving the environment, holding on to the physiological and psychological response, and storing it to equip oneself in the future should they experience a similar situation again (Touro University, 2016). When an individual finds a situation to be unpleasant, they are likely to avoid similar situations in the future. In some cases, emotional suffering may occur because of the ongoing experience avoidance. By averting oneself, psychological rigidity manifests and the individual is unable to behave in accordance with their own core values.

Ten-year-old Bradly rather enjoyed going to church on Sunday. He enjoyed the worship time and connecting to his environment. One year, Bradly went to the youth group summer camp for a week. While he was there, they had a Bible competition. The boys were given a Bible verse and told to find it in the text as quickly as possible. Those that found the verse the fastest, were given points for their cabin. Bradly was new to the Bible and didn't know how to look up verses very well. Ultimately, he was the slowest one in his group of boys. The boys berated him for being slow. When Bradly returned home, he never wanted to look up verses in the Bible again. In fact, he rather despised the book. Bradly's core value of spiritual connection had been affected. His avoidance of reading the Bible conflicted with his core value of a relationship with God. Rather than challenging negative thoughts, ACT works on acceptance, mindfulness, cognitive diffusion, values and committed action to reach a therapeutic end point. In Bradly's case, accepting that he was new to the Bible, being mindful spiritual connection is about more than a Bible verse competition, being committed to returning to his core value of spiritual connection, and having behavioral skills to assist his desire for change could ultimately lead him to a new view his relationship with God.

Family Therapy

In my years as a physician, I can only think of a handful of cases where individual therapy was "enough" for a child. Your youngster will be far more successful if you engage in treatment alongside them. Family therapy helps parents and their children nurture change and development. It is a safe place for family members to communicate while an unbiased licensed specialist facilitates the session. Family therapy can be done intermittently with your child's therapist; however, I strongly recommend an alternative counselor to serve in this role.

When my daughter turned 14 years old, she started down a very unhealthy path. The combination of adolescence, parent divorce, and a global pandemic was the perfect storm. Drastic measures were needed to get my child back on the path to success. If she had done treatment alone, there would not have been enough change in the family unit to support what she required.

Being a parent can be humbling. Despite my years of training in the medical profession, I acknowledged I did not have the skills needed to help my child. Her success ultimately depended on a team-based approach including her pediatrician, an adolescent therapist, a psychiatrist, and an educational specialist. While she was working hard in her sessions, I took accompanying parenting classes, which subsequently led to a great deal of my own homework. I also participated actively in parent support groups and family counseling sessions.

In working alongside my children as they achieve emotional wellbeing, I have found it useful having my own therapist, as they have theirs. When everyone has their own provider to engage with it makes it easier to be open and honest. There is more fulfillment from the therapeutic sessions. When my child and I have required family therapy, I have engaged a behavioral consultant separate from our own providers. This has helped mediate discussion without any one individual feeling like the therapist is biased towards one party or another. To better facilitate conversation, I sign consent forms so that all the providers can discuss our case separate from our sessions in hopes of overall achieving a more cohesive family unit.

Animal Assisted Therapy (AAT)

As a Doctor of Osteopathic Medicine, I understand the need to care for my patients as an integrated whole, rather than to treat for specific symptoms. To treat my patient's body, mind, and soul, I have frequently utilized complementary therapy techniques. Animal Assisted Therapy (AAT) describes a complementary intervention with animals, generally dogs, which have been trained to be obedient, calm, and comforting (Marcus et. al, 2012). AAT has been found to be acceptable and useful to optimize healing environments. In fact, several publications evaluating the benefits of AAT visits suggest 10-15 minutes of interaction improves patient wellbeing across a wide range of medical conditions (Marcus et. al, 2012).

Interactions with animals have been a favorite human pursuit since the beginning of time. Animals possess qualities that mark them as uniquely suited to be a healing companion as they are loyal, loving, and readily available creatures (Machova et. al, 2019). AAT has shown beneficial results in psychotherapy as the presence of an animal can reduce the activity of the sympathetic nervous system (the pathway of the body that puts all your senses in alert mode) (Marcus et. al, 2013). I happily include Ranger, an adorable golden retriever, in my practice encounters. Adding Ranger to my office improved both patient and staff satisfaction. In fact, I have patients who only like to schedule appointments on "Ranger Office Days." I also have patients who have come to the office to establish care because they heard I supplemented with AAT.

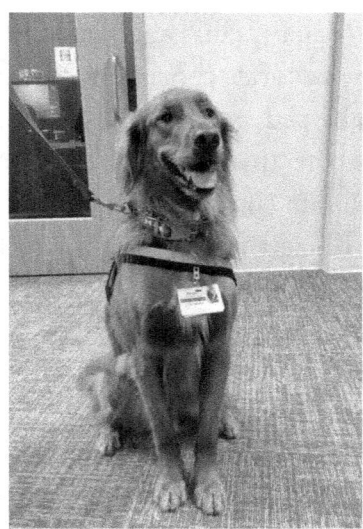

Dr. Ranger, DOG

<u>Summary</u>

Therapy is more than lying on a sofa telling a medical professional how you feel. Therapy is the attempted remediation of a health problem, often following a medical diagnosis. As a rule, each type of therapy has an indication, as well as a contraindication. Not all therapies are effective for all individuals. The goal of treatment is for your child to develop positive thinking and coping skills to treat the daily human challenges they face. Schools focus on mathematics, science, history, and language arts but do not have the time to focus on emotional regulation. This is where you as a parent can step in and be sure your child has the tools they need to become productive and well-adjusted.

Homework: Learn and practice emotional regulation techniques. (Additional Matter – Your Story).

Chapter 7

MEDICATIONS & SUPPLEMENTS

When it comes to starting children on medication management, I typically see one of three different situations in my medical practice. Many parents are anxious when it comes to putting their child on medication management. I can understand this hesitancy. The human brain continues to develop until an individual is approximately 25 years of age (Arain et. al, 2013). There are several chemical reactions that occur in the adolescent body as a child grows to set the stage for the "adult brain." The last part of brain development is the frontal lobe (Arain et. al, 2013). The frontal lobe is essential for executive tasks, such as planning, working memory, and impulse control. It is understandable parents would be concerned about the addition of "foreign" materials, such as medication or supplementation, to the developing mind.

A second set of parents that come to my office are those who would prefer to place their child on medication to "fix their behavior" or to "make them listen." Despite their belief that medication has this potential, there is no "perfect child pill." Medications do not change the core of an individual. They do not make up for the environment the child is surrounded by at home or at school. Medications will not address inconsistent parenting, lack of exercise, excessive technology exposure, bullying at school, or poor self-image. Wellness takes work. A child's recovery from mental illness needs a comprehensive team of individuals cooperating to support the youngster's needs. The squad may consist of the child, parents, teacher, counselor, and physician. The group may need the child, parents, behavioral therapist, occupational therapist, counselor, physician, psychiatrist, school staff, and clergy. There is no one-size-fits-all approach to mental health.

A third set of parents I encounter are somewhere in the middle. While they are uneasy about the idea of starting their youngster on medication, they understand supplementation, whether through pharmaceuticals or vitamins, may be necessary. Neurophysiology is complex. The brain is not static (Arain et. al, 2013). When I talk to patients about medication management as it relates to mental health I focus on the chemical imbalance. Adolescence is the time when children become adults. This period is full of change, both gonadal and behavioral. The limbic system is the part of the brain that is involved in behavioral response (Smith, 2015). This system helps to facilitate memory storage and retrieval, establish emotional states, and link the conscious functions of the brain with the unconscious functions of the brain. During puberty, the increases in estrogen and testosterone bind receptors in the limbic system, which not only stimulates sex drive, but also increase adolescents' emotional volatility and impulsivity (Arain et. al, 2013).

In a brain under stress, the limbic system is activated in a way that damages the body. Long term release of stress hormones can damage blood vessels, cause blood pressure to increase, and change appetite. In this way, stress can kill brain cells and even reduce the size of the brain (Touro University, 2016). Chronic tension can have a long-lasting effect on the prefrontal cortex, the area of the brain responsible for memory and learning.

When a medication is prescribed to a patient, the physician does so by looking at the benefits of clinical response compared to the risks of side effects from the medication. Psychiatric medications influence the brain chemicals that regulate thought patterns. Ideally, children would be successful participating solely in therapeutic sessions and learning emotional regulation techniques. In some cases, mental health symptoms may be so significant they interfere with the therapeutic plan. Adding medication may be helpful in reducing symptoms so psychotherapy may be more effective. Medications do not create an artificial form of wellness (Peterson, 2019). They balance abnormal chemistry in the brain that has occurred due to unfortunate conditions.

The best way to learn about a prescription your child has been given is by reviewing the package insert that accompanies the medication. For every drug on the market, pharmaceutical companies are required to develop a product monograph that is approved by the national regulatory agency and includes dosing of the medication, possible drug interactions, and potential side effects (Peterson, 2019). Psychiatric medications may have beneficial or adverse interactions with other prescription medications, over-the-counter drugs, supplements, vitamins, and herbs. It is important to let your physician know everything your child is taking, whether prescribed by a provider or not. It is also crucial the provider knows all the health problems, including drug allergies and intolerances, your child has been diagnosed with previously.

A few words of caution. First, potential side effects listed by the drug company include any poor reaction experienced by an individual during previous medication clinical trials or ongoing after-market surveillances (Peterson, 2019). These symptoms may, or may not, be related to the drug alone. Looking at the list of side effects does not give you complete information to make an informed decision on the treatment by itself. Drug companies are likely to err on the side of publishing more, not less, possible symptoms to avoid lawsuits later (Peterson, 2019). Second, knowing everything you can about a medication does not tell you how your child's body will respond to the medication. There are genetic blood tests which may be ordered by your youngster's provider to determine which medications are more easily metabolized by their body, but even those cannot predict adverse events. This unpredictability of treatment may be one reason psychiatry medication has developed an unfortunate stigma. Being knowledgeable about pharmaceuticals and supplementation can help lead you to making the right decision for your child.

"Will my child have to take this medication for the rest of their life?" This is a very common question parents ask when we start discussing medication management in my office. My response is almost always, "That depends." Recall that medications alone do not equal wellness. If a child starts on medication management, participates in the appropriate behavioral interventions, but the environment which caused the discord does not change, then the likelihood of the abnormal brain chemistry returns, leading to higher potential for mental illness relapse. The child will be more likely to remain on medication, or even need additional doses of medication over time.

I cannot stress the importance of a team-based approach to your child's wellness enough. The programs in which my children have been the most successful in obtaining optimal health have been the programs where medication was a small part of the overall big picture. I have spent hundreds of hours participating in parent support groups and family therapy sessions and reading books or journals to support my child. If your child had cancer, you'd likely learn as much as you could about the disease and perform a long search for the best oncology group. Your child's depression or anxiety is no different. Their long-term success is based on your means to help them find the right resources when they cannot.

Drug Basics

Take a deep breath. In and out. Relax your shoulders. Breathe again, once more. Slowly. Is your mind clear? If not, try it again. There is no way to sugar coat a chapter on medication and supplements and make it an exciting read. I am a nerd and proud of it. I find it exciting to read medical texts and learn new concepts and challenge my mind. Despite this fact, even I cannot get through a fact-based pharmaceutical book without a cup of coffee and a stretch break… or four.

A thorough description of neurophysiology and drug metabolism is out of the scope for this book. If you're interested in a deeper dive into the topic, I'd like to refer you to *Psych Meds Made Simple: How & Why They Do What They Do*, written by Ashley L. Peterson. Ms. Peterson's first career was as a pharmacist, but she chose to give that up to become a nurse and found her calling in mental health. For the purpose of this text, I believe a brief synopsis is sufficient.

The human brain is made up of billions of nerve cells called neurons (Peterson, 2019). Neurons communicate through chemical messengers, known as neurotransmitters. Neurotransmitters are passed from one cell to another to act on specific receptors on the nerve cell membrane (Peterson, 2019). This behavior passes along a signal. There are a variety of neurotransmitters that act throughout the brain to accomplish a variety of functions. When it comes to mental illness, there are some chemical messengers that are more relevant than others, specifically: serotonin, norepinephrine, dopamine, GABA, and glutamate (Peterson, 2019). Medications that boost a receptor's normal activity are called agonists. Medications that block receptors to prevent neurotransmitters from doing their normal thing are called antagonists, or blockers (Peterson, 2019).

Neurotransmitters and What They Do	
Serotonin	<ul><li>Mood stabilizer</li><li>Helps with digestion</li><li>Low levels lead to increased depression, high anxiety, and poor sleep quality</li></ul>
Norepinephrine	<ul><li>Increases arousal and attention</li><li>Low levels lead to lack of energy and reduced concentration</li></ul>
Dopamine	<ul><li>Allows feelings of pleasure, satisfaction, and motivation</li><li>Low levels lead to depression, too high levels lead to mania, and impulse control</li></ul>
GABA	<ul><li>Natural brain relaxant</li><li>Low levels lead to increased stress and anxiety</li></ul>
Glutamate	<ul><li>An amino acid in the brain that has an excitatory effect</li><li>Low levels lead to concentration difficulty, mental exhaustion, and insomnia</li></ul>

Different areas of the brain are responsible for alternative functions, even if they communicate using the same neurotransmitters. The goal of treatment may be to target a certain receptor in each portion of the brain, but medications are not that specific. Effecting the neurotransmitters in one area may cause unwanted effects in another region. Neurotransmitters also interplay with one another to create downstream effects. For this reason, it is not as easy as increase neurotransmitter "X" or decrease neurotransmitter "Y."

When medications are taken by mouth, they are absorbed through the gastrointestinal lining. The chemicals then move into the bloodstream and travel to the location of effect. For some drugs, absorption depends on how the medication is consumed, for instance, whether it is taken with food (Peterson, 2019). If extended-release tablets are split or chewed, this can interfere with their time releasing properties. Medications covered with an enteric coating are dissolved by the body further along the gastrointestinal tract to prevent stomach upset. An individual's metabolism may be affected by genetics, other medications, hydration status, or illnesses that target specific organs (e.g., stomach, intestine, liver, or kidneys) (Peterson, 2019). There are also medications that have a narrow therapeutic window, meaning there is a small concentration range between the drug having a positive effect and a toxic outcome (Peterson, 2019). Lithium, for instance, is one of these medications and should have regular blood testing to be sure an individual remains safe during treatment.

Every drug has a generic name and a chemical name. When a medication first comes to market, it is given a patent by the U.S. Food and Drug Administration. For many pharmaceuticals this patent lasts 20 years (U.S. Food & Drug Administration, 2020). During this time, only the original manufacturer can produce the medication. When a patent expires, other companies may produce their own version of the medication. These formulations are known as generics. Generic drugs are carefully created to have the same quality, safety, and effectiveness as the brand name drug. Generic medications are nearly always less expensive than the parent brand drug.

Some patients feel the generic version of the medication does not work the same as the brand name product they were originally prescribed. Generics are required to have the same active ingredients, in the same amount, as the original. However, other ingredients in the pill, such as fillers, can be different. A filler is an inactive substance used to make active medicine easier to measure (Stoppler, 2021). For example, fillers are often used in tablets or capsules because the amount of active drug is too small to be handled conveniently. Fillers can alter how the medications is absorbed by the body.

Drugs have different potencies. In other words, different amounts of similar medications may be required to have an equivalent effect (Peterson, 2019). Dosages are expressed by their units of measurement. Medications with large amounts (measured in grams, g) have less potency. Medications with smaller amounts (measured in micrograms, mcg) have higher potency. Medications somewhere in the middle are measured in milligrams, mg. It is not helpful to make a judgement about a medication, or its effectiveness, based solely on a number given for its dose (Peterson, 2019). It is more meaningful to look up the dosing range of a particular medication and see how the dose prescribed compares to that range. A high dose may mean increased effectiveness of the medication. Unfortunately, an elevated dose may come with increased side effects (Peterson, 2019).

Some parents have expressed concern to me that they are fearful of their child becoming "addicted" to psychiatric medications. If a medication is used to manage mental health symptoms, and then the drug is discontinued and symptoms return, this does not represent addiction (Peterson, 2019) If I prescribed a patient with diabetes insulin, and their blood sugars improved, and then insulin was stopped and their blood sugars increased again, we wouldn't think the patient was "addicted to insulin." Psychiatric supplementation is no different. Chronic ailments are often managed by specific treatments. Sometimes treatments are curative, but in most cases, the illness is likely to become uncontrolled again if the treatment is eliminated from the picture.

Tolerance of a medication occurs when an individual takes a medication for a period and the body begins to require higher doses of the substance to achieve the same effect it had as the original dose (Peterson, 2019). Tolerance does not occur with all medications, or with all individuals. Tolerance is more common with some medications than others. Benzodiazepines used for anxiety is a good example. Christina scheduled an appointment in my office because her clonazepam (Klonopin) "stopped working." She was taking 0.25mg twice daily and this had helped for five years. Now when Christina took 0.25mg of clonazepam she did not have any improvement in her symptoms. When she took 0.5mg of clonazepam her anxiety returned to baseline. Christina's body had become tolerant of her previously prescribed treatment. In situations such as these, it's common for me to prescribe a "drug holiday." During a drug holiday, I prescribe an alternative medication to help the patient for 3-4 weeks while their body becomes less resistant to the original treatment. When I restart the original medication a month later, frequently the patient finds the medication beneficial again.

The purpose of this chapter is not to serve as a pharmacopeia with a list of medicinal drugs and their many uses, preparations, dosages, and formulas. Instead, I wish to introduce you to key medication players in mental health. Should your healthcare provider introduce the concept of medication management for your child, I want you to be confident in your treatment decision. Going forward, let's explore the different classifications of psychiatric medications and supplements.

Anti-Depressant Medications

The most common medications used to treat depression are the *selective serotonin reuptake inhibitors (SSRIs)*. SSRIs became popular in the late 1980s with the introduction of fluoxetine (Prozac). Before SSRIs, monoamine oxidase inhibitors (MAOIs) and tricyclic antidepressants (TCAs) were the mainstay of treatment. While MAOIs and TCAs were effective, they were known to have significant undesirable side effects. SSRIs inhibit serotonin reuptake on the pre-synaptic (nerve firing) side of nerve cell communication (Peterson, 2019). As a result, there is more serotonin floating around, ready to bind with receptors on the post-synaptic (nerve accepting) neuron. The increased availability of serotonin occurs quickly, but the downregulation of receptors ready to accept the serotonin occurs a little slower (Peterson, 2019). The "selective" part of the SSRI name means that while much of the drug's activity is directly on serotonin transporters, most of the SSRIs have effects at other receptors causing slight variations in how they work and the potential for wanted, or unwanted, side effects.

Common SSRIs	
Fluoxetine (Prozac)	Fluvoxamine (Luvox)
Sertraline (Zoloft)	Paroxetine (Paxil)
Citalopram (Celexa)	Escitalopram (Lexapro)
Vilazodone (Viibryd)	Vortioxetine (Trintellix)

Side effects of SSRIs are related to increased serotonin activity in the brain and in the gastrointestinal tract. In my experience, side effects are worse when first starting an SSRI or increasing the dose as it takes an individual time to adjust to the increased presence of serotonin. Potential side effects include, but are not limited to headache, fatigue, poor sleep, sweating, dizziness, dry mouth, nausea, vomiting, abdominal cramping, or diarrhea (Peterson, 2019). There may be weight gain, though I have only witnessed this to be upwards of five pounds in most individuals. Too much serotonin may cause lack of interest or enthusiasm and the dose may need to be reduced.

Serotonin syndrome is a condition when there is excessive activation of serotonin in the brain (Peterson, 2019). When an individual gets too much of the neurotransmitter, they can significantly suffer. Individuals with serotonin syndrome generally go to the hospital with concerns of headache, confusion, hallucinations, sweating, fever, increased blood pressure and heart rate, nausea, vomiting, and involuntary muscle contractions (Mayo Clinic, 2022). I am always aware of the possibility of serotonin syndrome. As a physician, I am cautious when prescribing medications that can boost the effects of an SSRI. Usually, if prescribers are aware of all medications, supplements, and vitamins an individual is taking and the individual takes medications as prescribed, serotonin syndrome can be avoided in most cases.

Another class of medication used to treat depression is *serotonin and norepinephrine reuptake inhibitors (SNRIs)*. SNRIs have a similar effect to SSRIs, but they also inhibit reuptake of norepinephrine. Norepinephrine reuptake transporters are responsible not just for their effects on the neurotransmitter norepinephrine, but also for recycling the neurotransmitter, dopamine. This means that an SNRI may end up affecting the regulation of dopamine as well. Specific SNRIs may have a preferential for acting more on serotonin or more on norepinephrine.

In some medications, the preferential is determined based on the dose of the drug.

Common SNRIs	
Venlafaxine (Effexor)	Desvenlafaxine (Pristiq)
Duloxetine (Cymbalta)	Levomilnacipran (Fetzima)

Potential side effects of SNRIs include tremor, increased heart rate, and increased blood pressure (Peterson, 2019). These symptoms often present when starting a medication or titrating the dose of the medication but may not last. Other side effects may include dry mouth, constipation, urinary retention, and changes in vision (Peterson, 2019). These side effects may be less likely to improve with persistent use of the medication. Due to the serotonin component of these medications, SNRIs may cause nausea and increased anxiety.

There is only one norepinephrine and dopamine reuptake inhibitor (NDRI) currently on the market, bupropion (Wellbutrin). There is a small risk of seizure activity when this medication is administered. This risk is elevated at higher doses of the medication and with alcohol consumption. Since electrolyte abnormalities can occur with individuals suffering from eating disorders that include purging, the seizure risk is also elevated in these individuals. Other side effects include dry mouth, blurred vision, constipation, urinary retention, and insomnia (Peterson, 2019).

Tricyclic antidepressants (TCAs) are an older group of medications. These drugs block the reuptake of serotonin and norepinephrine, but not in a clean fashion like the SNRIs (Peterson, 2019). TCAs are known to have considerable side effects such as lack of energy, weight gain, low blood pressure, dry mouth, constipation, urinary retention, seizures, and abnormal heart rhythms. TCAs may be potentially lethal in an overdose (Peterson, 2019). I do not regularly prescribe TCAs to pediatric patients.

Common TCAs	
Amitriptyline (Elavil)	Imipramine (Tofranil)
Clomipramine (Anafranil)	Doxepin (Silenor)
Desipramine (Norpramin)	Nortriptyline (Pamelor)

Monoamine oxidase inhibitors (MAOIs) boost neurotransmitter signally of serotonin, norepinephrine, and dopamine (Peterson, 2019). This is also an older class of medications and known to have significant side effects. In the gastrointestinal system, the enzyme MAO-A is responsible for breaking down an amino acid, tyramine. Individuals on MAOIs are unable to metabolize tyramine. Tyramine is contained in foods like smoked meat, aged cheese, soy, tofu, and draft beer (Peterson, 2019). If tyramine does not get broken down and absorbed into the blood stream, a dangerously high blood pressure known as hypertensive crisis can result. There is a different kind of MAOI known as a reversible inhibitor of MAO-A (RIMA). Moclobemide (Manerix) is an example of this type of medication. It does not completely block MAO-A in the gut (Peterson, 2019). Nevertheless, there are many potential drug interactions with this class of medications (e.g., migraine medications, cough suppressant and some decongestants). MAOIs may also cause weight gain, swelling, disordered sleep, orthostatic hypotension, and muscle pain (Peterson, 2019). I do not regularly prescribe MAOIs to pediatric patients.

Trazodone (Desyrel) is an antagonist at two serotonin receptors and acts as a serotonin reuptake inhibitor (Peterson, 2019). It acts as an antidepressant in high doses, but it is seldom used for this purpose due to its intolerability at these doses. Most often, trazodone is used as a sleep aid due to its sedative effects. I have found trazodone to be an effective medication to help pediatrics suffering with insomnia.

Anxiolytic Medications (Anti-Anxiety Medications)

A genetic variation in the gene encoding for the serotonin reuptake transporter has been associated with an increased susceptibility for experiencing fear in response to external stressors (Peterson, 2019). SSRIs, therefore, have been found useful in the treatment of anxiety. Improvement in anxiety is heavily dependent on changes in the serotonin receptor regulation and sensitivity. This takes time. It may take four to six weeks to see a reduction in anxiety after a medication has been initiated. SSRIs may worsen anxiety while it takes time for the receptors to adapt. These medications are often started at lower doses and titrated slowly to avoid this undesirable effect. I will sometimes prescribe short-term use of benzodiazepines to manage a patient's symptoms when they are first introduced to an SSRI.

Gamma-aminobutyric acid (GABA) is a calming neurotransmitter in the brain (Cuncic, 2022). GABA is made up of various subunits. A medication interacting with the neurotransmitter will demonstrate a different effect depending on the subunit acted on. Alcohol and benzodiazepines affect the GABA mechanism (Peterson, 2019). Benzodiazepines are sedating and are often used for acute agitation, sedation before medical procedures, anxiety, or sleep (Peterson, 2019). While they are effective for short-term use, long-term use is generally not recommended due to their addictive potential. Short-term side effects may include sedation, confusion, and poor memory. Long-term side effects include tolerance and dependence (Peterson, 2019). Tolerance was previously discussed so I will focus on dependence.

Common Benzodiazepines	
Alprazolam (Xanax)	Clonazepam (Klonopin)
Diazepam (Valium)	Lorazepam (Ativan)
Temazepam (Restoril)	

There are two types of dependence: psychological and physiological (Peterson, 2019). Psychological dependence is the person's belief the medication is necessary to function. Without the medication, they cannot complete day-to-day activities. Physiological dependence is demonstrated when an individual abruptly discontinues a medication, and it produces withdrawal symptoms. Examples of withdrawal from benzodiazepines involve muscle cramps, changes in heart rate, changes in blood pressure, anxiety, agitation, trouble sleeping, impaired memory and hallucinations (Peterson, 2019). To prevent withdrawal, benzodiazepines need to be tapered very slowly. In patients that have been on this type of medication for several years, it can take a very long time to wean off the medication, if it is even possible. I do not recommend benzodiazepines as long-term therapy in children.

Beta blockers are medications that work outside the brain to slow the body down. One beta blocker, propranolol (Inderal) has been used for performance anxiety, such as nervousness when giving a speech or taking a test. Other uses for this medication are to control blood pressure, heart rate, or for migraine prevention. I do not recommend this class of medications for individuals with asthma as they can increase spasms within the lungs.

Buspirone (Buspar) is a partial agonist at serotonin receptors (Peterson, 2019). It ultimately allows for more time for regeneration of serotonin in the neuron. Buspirone can take up to six weeks to take effect. However, I have many patients who utilize buspirone as needed up to three times daily and do very well managing their anxiety. While typical dosage is 20 to 30mg daily divided into two to three doses, I have found even 5mg can be effective. For pediatric patients with more anxiety symptoms than depressive symptoms, I have noticed this to be a good fit.

Two antihistamines are commonly used to treat anxiety. Hydroxyzine (Atarax) is an antihistamine that influences serotonin. Diphenhydramine (Benadryl, Unisom) is an antihistamine that is sedating and used to help with insomnia. I have encountered youngsters who pick at their skin and believe it to be "itchy," especially in times of high stress. Hydroxyzine may be useful for these individuals. A word of caution about diphenhydramine: In young children this can have a paradoxical effect, meaning, the effect of the medication is the opposite of what would usually be expected. For diphenhydramine, the effect may be hyperactivity instead of sedation.

Mood Stabilizers

Bipolar disorder is associated with a chemical imbalance involving several neurotransmitters. Mood stabilizers have complex effects on nerve signaling cascades (Peterson, 2019). Many mood stabilizers induce side effects at high doses. For this reason, if an individual is having some improvement on a mood stabilizer at a moderate dose but continues to exhibit some highs and lows of mania and depression, combination therapy with another medication group is frequently utilized (Peterson, 2019). It should be noted mood stabilizers are known to have interactions with other medications and this may limit their ultimate use. When an individual is on two medications known to interact with one another, they may require frequent provider monitoring and possibly extra laboratory testing.

Common Mood Stabilizers	
Lithium	Valproic Acid (Depakote)
Carbamazepine (Tegretol)	Lamotrigine (Lamictal)

Lithium has been used as a treatment for bipolar for many years. It works in the brain by boosting the calming neurotransmitter GABA (Peterson, 2019). Lithium enhances the effects of antidepressants in the treatment of major depressive disorders. It is known to reduce the risk of suicide (Peterson, 2019). Lithium is metabolized by the kidneys. If an individual is dehydrated, the kidneys cannot functionally optimally, and this lowers the threshold for lithium toxicity. Lithium has a narrow therapeutic window. Frequent blood testing is required to ensure safety on the medication. When I order blood work on individuals prescribed lithium, I ask to have their labs drawn 12 hours following the last medication dose to get the most accurate test result. Blood work includes checking electrolytes (such as sodium, potassium), kidney function, and lithium level. If lithium dosing needs to be adjusted, it typically takes five days for blood levels to stabilize (Peterson, 2019).

Symptoms of mild lithium toxicity are tremor, impaired concentration, confusion, and loose stools. Irregular heartbeat, seizures and coma may result from more severe lithium toxicity. Side effects from lithium levels in range may include hair loss, dizziness, weight gain, acne, sedation, dry mouth, metallic taste, frequent urination, and increased thirst. Lithium also interferes with the production of thyroid hormones leading to hypothyroidism (Peterson, 2019).

Valproic acid (Depakote) and carbamazepine (Tegretol) should also have regular laboratory monitoring. For valproic acid it is common to check electrolytes, kidney function, liver function, and valproic acid level. For carbamazepine, since it may influence bone marrow development, I order a complete blood count to look at blood cells, platelets, and other cells found in the blood in addition to liver function tests and carbamazepine levels. Side effects of valproic acid and carbamazepine are like lithium. Valproic acid can cause nausea, sedation, weight gain, hair loss, and tremor. Carbamazepine side effects include sedation, dizziness, impaired coordination, dry mouth, constipation, urinary retention, and blurred vision (Peterson, 2019).

Most frequently, I prescribe lamotrigine (Lamictal) for mood stabilization. Lamotrigine must be started at low doses and increased slowly. Lamotrigine does have side effects of dizziness, headache, double vision, nausea, dry mouth, and weight gain, but it tends to be tolerated much better than other mood stabilizers (Peterson, 2019). Laboratory testing is not monitored in the same fashion as other mood stabilizers. Skin reactions must be very closely monitored on lamotrigine and the medication discontinued if an adverse event occurs.

Anti-Psychotics

While the name "anti-psychotic" sounds intimidating, the medications in this class are used for a variety of conditions aside from psychotic disorders. Atypical antipsychotics are often used in bipolar disorder and sometimes major depressive disorder. All anti-psychotics act by blocking dopamine receptors (Peterson, 2019). The "typical" antipsychotics are an older generation of the medication classification and may have more side effects than the newer "atypical" medication counterparts. First- generation anti-psychotics caused extrapyramidal events (inability to sit still, involuntary muscle contraction, tremors, stiff muscles, and involuntary facial movements) (Purse, 2022). Side effects of second-generation anti-psychotics are more in line with weight gain leading to increased risk of high cholesterol and diabetes.

First-Generation Anti-Psychotics	
Haloperidol (Haldol)	Loxapine (Loxapac)
Zuclopenthixol (Clopixol)	Fluphenazine (Prolixin, Modecate)
Flupenthixol (Fluanxol)	
Second-Generation Anti-Psychotics	
Clozapine (Clozaril)	Olanzapine (Zyprexa)
Risperidone (Risperdal)	Paliperidone (Invega)
Quetiapine (Seroquel)	Sulpiride (Dogmatil)
Ziprasidone (Zeldox, Geodon)	Aripiprazole (Abilify)
Lurasidone (Latuda)	Asenapine (Saphris)
Cariprazine (Vraylar)	Brexpiprazole (Rexulti)

Stimulants

Attention-deficit/hyperactivity disorder (ADHD) involves deficits in attention and executive functioning. In ADHD, there is an imbalance in the neurotransmitters norepinephrine and dopamine (Peterson, 2019). Many parents become concerned when I talk about adding stimulant medication for their hyperactive child. They may believe stimulants to be like the caffeine in their morning coffee and fear waking up their already hyperactive child. Stimulants do "wake up the brain," but they do this by increasing the activity to the lacking chemical signals that are meant to improve focus and impulse control. Stimulants work for the day they are taken. When administering medication to your child, you will typically see results within 30 to 60 minutes.

Stimulants	
Dextroamphetamine (Adderall)	Lisdexamfetamine (Vyvanse)
Methylphenidate (Ritalin, Concerta)	

Side effects of stimulants include weight loss, dry mouth, insomnia, anxiety, dizziness, stomach upset, rapid heart rate, elevated blood pressure, and restlessness (Peterson, 2019). When used in the pediatric population, it can stunt growth so frequent visits with the healthcare provider (at least every three months) are crucial for drug monitoring. Because of concerns about growth, many parents opt out of giving their children stimulants on weekends, holidays, or school breaks when attention and academic performance is less crucial.

Atomoxetine (Strattera) is a selective norepinephrine reuptake inhibitor. It does not affect dopamine. Side effects are similar to the stimulant class of medication (headache, loss of appetite, increased blood pressure, increased heart rate, and mood swings) (Peterson, 2019). Unlike stimulants where the effect is felt for the day the medication is taken, atomoxetine must build up in the body over at least four weeks before maximum effectiveness and must be taken daily.

Vitamins and Dietary Supplementation

I firmly believe in the benefits of vitamins and dietary supplementation in the world of mental health. I commonly prescribe over the counter supplements as adjunctive treatment for my patients. If your child is on medication management for mental health, vitamins and supplements should be administered with caution and under the guidance of a healthcare profession. Some remedies, while easily available at the local supermarket or online, may interfere with the metabolic pathway of the prescription medication. In most cases, I order laboratory testing to look for deficiencies before making a recommendation for complementary therapy. Below are examples of items I commonly use in my integrative medicine practice.

Vitamins and Supplements	
5-HTP	5-HTP supplements are thought to treat depression by increasing serotonin levels (Greenblatt & Lee, 2019).
Acetyl-L-Carnitine	Important nutrient derived from amino acids, Tyrosine and Methionine. Helps with synthesis of DHA which is critical for healthy brain development. Low carnitine is associated with behavioral problems (Greenblatt & Lee, 2019).
GABA	GABA is an inhibitory neurotransmitter. GABA calms the brain and slows down the central nervous system. It may be helpful to treat anxiety (Cuncic, 2022).
Glutamate	Glutamate is an excitatory neurotransmitter. Too little glutamate may lead to difficulty concentrating, insomnia, or mental exhaustion (Greenblatt & Lee, 2019).
Folic Acid	Folate supplements may reduce symptoms of treatment-resistant depression in children who have a genetic mutation that affects folate metabolism (Greenblatt & Lee, 2019).
Iron	Individuals with iron deficiency have an increased risk for anxiety, depression, sleep disorders, and psychotic disorders (Berzin, 2018).
Kava Kava	Kava is best known for its relaxing qualities. Kava is said to elevate mood, wellbeing, and contentment, and produce feelings of relaxation (Mount Sinai, 2022).

L-Theanine	L-theanine is a relaxing agent thought to relieve stress and anxiety (Wu, 2016).
Magnesium Glycinate	Magnesium has a calming effect on the body. Low magnesium can lead to anxiety, inattention, and poor sleep quality (Greenblatt & Gottlieb, 2017).
Melatonin	Melatonin is used by individuals struggling to get adequate sleep. It must be used cautiously as it can cause sleep dependency, fatigue, and worsen depressive symptoms (Greenblatt & Lee, 2019).
N-acetylcysteine (NAC)	NAC is a precursor to the amino acids L-cysteine and glutathione. Glutathione helps regulate oxidative damage in the body and provides anti-inflammatory benefits. NAC may improve neurotransmitter dysregulation (Kubala, 2021).
Omega	Omega 3 may support proper brain flow to the brain and therefore improve performance on cognitive tasks (Better Fish, 2020).
Phosphatidylserine	Phospholipid is made from the amino acid, Serine. Supports memory, mood, attention and the ability to communicate (Glade & Smith, 2015).
Pycnogenol	An extract from the bark of the French maritime pine that has antioxidant and anti-inflammatory properties. Thought to decrease stress hormones (Greenblatt & Gottlieb, 2017).
S-adenosylmethionine (SAMe)	SAMe is a sulfuric containing compound. It has shown promise in the treatment of depression (Kubala, 2021).
St John's Wort	A popular herb that has shown promise in reducing symptoms of mild to moderate depression (Kubala, 2021).
Vitamin B6	Water-soluble vitamin. Helps with neurotransmitter synthesis in the brain (Kubala, 2021). Low vitamin B6 can lead to difficulty concentrating and short-term memory loss.
Vitamin B12	Vitamin B12 has been demonstrated to reduce depressive symptoms in people with depressive

	disorder when used adjunctively with an antidepressant medication (Kubala, 2021).
Vitamin C	Vitamin C is needed to convert tryptophan, an amino acid present in animal proteins, into serotonin. Individuals low in vitamin C may feel fatigued or depressed (Gupta, 2014).
Vitamin D	Vitamin D may reduce inflammation, regulate mood, and protect against neurocognitive dysfunction (Kubala, 2021).
Zinc	Zinc deficiency is strongly linked to an increased risk of depression and depression symptom severity (Kubala, 2021).

Stopping or Changing a Medication or Supplement

Some individuals experience a discontinuation syndrome when they stop taking a prescription medication (Peterson, 2019). This withdrawal syndrome can be very uncomfortable for those that are affected. Withdrawal is more likely to be seen when the medication is discontinued suddenly, rather than a gradual tapering of the medication. When a medicine is abruptly stopped the body does not have time to compensate for the change in neurotransmitter levels. Symptoms most commonly include nausea, diarrhea, poor sleep, muscle pain, anxiety, irritability, and dizziness (Peterson, 2019).

One third of my patients may improve on the first medication I prescribe to them. Some slight tweaking of medication dosage and they are good to go. Another third of my patients will never get maximum benefit from medications no matter which drug we utilize. These individuals may find enough improvement with a combination treatment from medications, supplements, and counseling to be able to function daily, but there will always be a struggle. The last third of patients may improve with medication but finding the right fit of treatment takes a couple of tries.

In patients where I am changing medication to fit their needs, I can stop one medication and start another the next day. I can wean completely down on a medication and discontinue it before starting another. Lastly, I can titrate down on one medication while titrating up another. This is called cross-titration. The way I decide to move from one medication to another depends on the medications involved and the patient. Changing from one SSRI, like citalopram (Celexa), to another SSRI, like sertraline (Zoloft) is generally well tolerated by most individuals. I'm more likely to stop one and start the other. If I have a patient moving from citalopram (Celexa) to venlafaxine (Effexor), I'm more likely to titrate down on the SSRI (citalopram) while titrating up on the SNRI (venlafaxine).

It would be great if one medication was all that was needed. Unfortunately, for a lot of individuals that is not the case. Combination therapy with one or more prescription medications or adding a prescription medication with a supplement is very common in mental health. Some medications when used together boost the effect of one another.

Evie is a 14-year-old who came to me because of symptoms of depression. I started fluoxetine 10mg once daily. When she returned in a month, she denied experiencing any side effects. She noted the medication helped her feel somewhat better, but she was still having more bad days than good days. I increased the dose to 20mg daily and saw her back again after three weeks. This time Evie mentioned her depression was better. She was having more good days than bad days, but her sleep was still an issue. Evie, her mother, and I discussed how to address sleep related issues. Evie appeared to have an adequate sleep hygiene routine before bed. My suggestions were to either add diphenhydramine (Benadryl, Unisom) at 25mg before bed, consider low dose melatonin between 3mg and 5mg daily before bed, start magnesium glycinate 200mg before bed, or add trazodone (Desyrel) 25mg once daily at bedtime. The three of us discussed the pros and cons of each choice. In the discussion, Evie admitted having intermittent anxiety which made it challenging to shut her mind off before bed. I recommended we try the magnesium approach. When Evie checked in a month later, she was feeling much better.

Finding the right combination of medication and supplementation for a youngster can be very frustrating for parents. There is a lot of trial and error. Understanding how medications work and possible side effects can help families make informed decisions. It is important to remember the beneficial effects of psychiatric medication often don't come immediately. Medications may need to be taken for an adequate period before dismissing them as ineffective. If after starting a medication or supplement you have questions or wonder if how your child is feeling is a side effect of the medication, please reach out to the prescribing physician.

Homework: Knowing what medications have been started and stopped, the dosages administered, and the reactions your child has had to various medications is extremely helpful when a prescriber is trying to determine a treatment plan. Keep a log of their medication management and bring it with you to all appointments. (Additional Matter – Medication Management).

Chapter 8

SIGN HERE! THE FAMILY CONTRACT

"Friday night after I get out of school, I am going to Sophia's," Olivia told her mother.

"Friday night is grandma's birthday party. You won't be able to see Sophia that day. The whole family is going to visit with her. Please come home right after school," her mother replied.

"Grandma has Alzheimer's. She won't know if I'm not there. Besides, old people's homes smell bad. I hate how awful her house smells," Olivia answered. "Sophia just got a new kitten. I've seen the pictures she's snapped. You can just pick me up after the party."

"That's not how it's going to go Olivia. Your grandmother will not be around forever. Your uncles, aunts and cousins will all be there. Family is important. I expect you to be at the party. I don't want to hear any more about this. You will spend time with your family, and you will act like you're enjoying it," Olivia's mother countered.

"I'm not going. I'm 16. I decide what I want to do and what I don't want to do. Not you!" Olivia shouted as she slammed her bedroom door. Olivia's mother followed in after her. Olivia had already flopped down on her bed, put in her AirPods, and cranked up Spotify.

"Oliva." Her mother tried to get her attention. "We aren't done with this conversation." She paused, waiting for Olivia to take out her earbuds. Nothing. "Oliva!!" her mother yelled.

Olivia paused her music. "What?"

"We were having a conversation and you stormed off."

"We were not having a conversation!" Olivia rolled her eyes. "I was experiencing a dictatorship," she said harshly.

"Can't we talk about this?" her mother asked.

"No need to. I'm going to Sophia's. You're going to grandma's birthday. Ta-da!"

"First, you're wrong. We are going to grandmother's party. Second, give me your phone. You've lost it for two days for arguing," her mother said sternly.

"What? The phone is mine, not yours. You can't just take it from me."

"The phone bill is paid by me, so the phone is my property. Hand it over." A clear battle of wills had been started between Olivia and her mother.

"UGH! You hate me! You never let me do anything! I can't wait to get out of here!" Olivia screamed as she threw her phone across the bed towards her mother.

Congratulations! You win! Yes, by the sheer fact that you are the parent, and they are the child, you win! What did you win? Every argument. Every challenge. Choices are yours when it comes to parenting. Now, I did not say every decision you make in parenting is the right one, mind you. Nonetheless, you win disagreements between you and your child. There is no need to argue with your offspring. Your child has spent the past several years being "them." You cannot out argue "them." "They" will always win in their eyes. Rather than argue, raise your voice, or get angry, what if the situation would have gone like this…

""Friday night after I get out of school, I am going to Sophia's," Olivia told her mother.

"Friday night is grandma's birthday party. You won't be able to see Sophia that day. The whole family is going to visit with her. Please come home right after school," her mother replied.

"Grandma has Alzheimer's. She won't know if I'm not there. Besides, old people's homes smell bad. I hate how awful her house smells," Olivia answered. "Sophia just got a new kitten. I've seen the pictures she's snapped. You can just pick me up after the party."

"Olivia, I hear you really enjoy spending time with your friend, Sophia, and you are really looking forward to seeing her new kitten. Your grandmother is getting older, and she will not have a lot more birthdays. I expect the party to last two hours. I recognize that you have been working hard at maintaining your grades, keeping your room clean, and helping with the dishes recently. After school, our family will celebrate with Grandma, but on the way home I will drop you off at Sophia's house. If her parents are okay with you spending the night, I can even pick you up the next morning."

"I really don't want to go to grandma's birthday," Olivia started, "But I guess I can go to Sophia's a little later. I'll see how long she's available Friday night."

I have made mistakes as a parent. As my children grew and became more independent, moving from elementary school through middle school to high school, whenever they challenged me, I thought I could get them to see my point of view. This generally led to a long dialogue of my child trying to prove they were correct, and me trying to show them why they were not. It was exhausting. Learning to communicate differently, and more effectively, with my child has changed our relationship.

Parenting is tough work. When your child was born, they did not come with an instruction manual to fit their individual needs. Moreover, having a child with mental health issues is like housing a volcano that can explode at any moment. Personally, I wish children came with a sign over their head that lit up saying "Warning! Outburst Coming!" accompanied with the emergency alert sound. By recognizing volcano eruptions as both a normal part of growing up and a part of mental disorders we can anticipate them and attempt to avoid the unpleasant feeling of surprise when they occur. Expectancy helps us to remain calm, not taking our child's comments personally, and not overreacting. Our children are in a constant state of flux. What our kids need most is for us to remain as stable as possible.

My medical career has taught me behavioral theory and treatment modalities. Being a parent has taught me it's not enough to have a set of philosophies. Parents need a toolbox: a set of skills that are practical and can address the specific habits, needs and concerns of each of their children. In earlier chapters, we explored various therapeutic and medication approaches. Incorporating the concept of the family contract I found to be extraordinarily helpful in bringing peace and unity within the home. When followed with consistency, the family contract is simple, direct, and can help relieve the tension you feel as a parent during a child's volcanic eruption.

A family contract is a written, signed agreement between parent(s) and child(ren) that outlines expectations to be completed. The contract also delineates consequences for failing to uphold the assigned responsibility. Why I fell in love with the family contract, is that it is a non-argumentative way for parents to clearly communicate expectations, allows children input into how they want to manage their tasks, and identifies the result that will occur when the child completes, or does not complete, their assignment. For example, within a family contract it may say "Ana will complete her homework by 5:00 p.m. every day after school in order to earn two hours of technology use." The parents' expectation is that Ana needs to complete her homework before she can have free time on electronics. Ana can give input as to a reasonable time the homework should be completed to achieve free time. The result, if Ana completes her homework by 5:00 p.m., then she gets to indulge in using her phone, computer, or gaming system. If Ana opts to procrastinate and is unable to accomplish her homework by 5:00 p.m., then she does not have access to her phone, computer, or gaming system. There is no argument between parent and child. The expectation was clear. If Ana does not earn technology time, it's on her for not completing her homework in a reasonable timeframe.

There are dozens of free family contract templates available online. Common family contracts include sibling peace agreements, pet care, homework completion, household chores, social media, cell phone use, and teen driving. Family contracts can be short and cover one topic, or long and cover many topics. Family contracts can be effectively utilized with preteens and adolescents. With the help of Homeward Bound, a nation-wide group of specialized therapists who support families of struggling teens, my family has successfully implemented family contracts. On the next page is one example of a family contract.

Our Family Contract

We hope our family will communicate directly. We commit to listening to one another and respecting one another's feelings. We will try to recognize the good in one another. We will be open and honest with one another. We will respond to one another in a non-reactive manner.

Family Interactions
In our family, individuals will...

1. Be willing to have a conversation.

2. Speak in a respectful tone.

3. Consider other's feelings.

4. Be accountable for our actions.

5. Respect one another's property, including asking before taking another's belongings.

Consequences of respectful behavior include:

1. Family members will have stronger relationships.

2. The home environment will be more enjoyable.

3. Individuals will be able to trust one another.

4. Children will be able to earn opportunities for privileges.

Consequences of disrespectful behavior include:

1. Family members will have a strained relationship.

2. The home environment will not be peaceful.

3. Individuals will lack trust with one another.

4. Children will lose privileges until relationships are repaired, respect has been reinstated, and trust has improved.

Personal Care
In our family, individuals will...

1. Make personal hygiene a priority (e.g., regularly showering, brushing teeth, changing clothing, brushing hair, and using deodorant).

2. Maintain a healthy lifestyle. Junk-like foods will be eaten in moderation.

3. Wear clothing as approved by the school dress code on school days and as approved by parent(s) on non-school days.

4. Participate in medical appointments, individual or family therapy sessions, or other events as scheduled by the parent(s).

5. Maintain bedtime at 10:00 p.m. on weekdays and 11:00 p.m. on weekends.

6. Maintain their bedrooms (e.g., keep living space tidy, wash and fold all laundry, take any dishes used to the kitchen sink).

Consequences for maintaining personal care:

1. Children will have improved physical health.

2. Children will have improved mental health.

3. Children will be more independent.

Consequences for not maintaining personal care:

1. Children will feel physically and mentally unwell.

2. If a child does not maintain adequate personal care, then the parent(s) will have a conversation with the child and a plan to get the child back on track will be made.

3. If the child continues to exhibit poor health choices, then the child may lose a privilege.

Academics
In our family, individuals will...

1. Participate fully in school, putting forth their best effort.

2. Avoid procrastinate on getting schoolwork completed.

3. Turn in homework on time.

4. Ask for help with assignments when needed.

Consequences when schoolwork is managed:

1. Managing coursework allows the child to be more independent.

2. Managing coursework helps build life skills.

3. Managing coursework opens the schedule to allow for more after-school and weekend opportunities.

4. Managing course work allows for more privileges, such as technology.

Consequences when schoolwork is not managed:

1. If the parent(s) have concerns over the child's coursework, a conversation will take place and a plan will be made to address the concern.

2. If coursework is not completed, a privilege may be withheld from the child until the coursework is completed.

3. If a consequence is given by the school, the child will fulfill the obligations of the school's consequence.

Cell Phone and Electronic Devices
In our family, individuals will...

1. Answer their phone/respond to text when contacted by the parent.

2. Turn in all usernames and passwords for any accounts to the parent(s).

3. Turn in their cellphone to be reviewed by parent(s) when asked.

4. Put away devices when asked (e.g., for mealtime, conservations, family, etc).

5. Turn off electronic devices by 9pm on school nights and 10pm on weekends.

6. Follow the school policy with regards to electronics in the classroom.

Consequences from following electronic guidelines:

1. Children will continue to have access to cell phones and other electronic devices.

2. Children will build trust by following the rules.

3. Children will be able to earn additional freedoms.

Consequences from not following electronic guidelines:

1. If a child refuses to put away their phone, respond to parents when called/texted, or does not allow a parent to view a device when asked, then the child will lose their device for a few hours to a few days.

2. If a child does not turn the device in on time at night, then they will lose an equal amount of time on the device the next day.

3. If any inappropriate material is posted or reviewed online or in text messages, the material will be removed from the device and access to electronics will be eliminated for one week.

4. If there are continued consequences resulting in loss of privileges to electronic devices, the parent(s) may remove electronic devices from the child for an indefinite period.

<u>Friends</u>

<u>In our family, individuals will...</u>

1. Introduce friends to the parent(s) and the parent(s) will get to know the friends before the child spends time with the friends outside of the home.

2. Be honest regarding their friends and their activities.

Consequences for following friend guidelines:

1. Children will continue to build new relationships.

2. Children will be able to earn more privileges regarding spending time with friends.

Consequences for not following friend guidelines:

1. The parent(s) will have a conversation with the child regarding their concerns and a plan will be made to help the child have healthier relationships and earn more trust.

2. If trust is lost with the child, it is likely that time with a particular friend may be lost or reduced until such time as trust can be earned again.

Requesting to Make Changes to the
Family Contract

A child may make a request to the parent(s) to addend the Family Contract. Before submitting the request, the child:

1. Will take the time to consider what concerns the parents may have with the request.

2. Be ready to suggest solutions to resolve parent concerns.

3. Given enough time for the child and the parent(s) to discuss the requested change.

The parent(s) will take time to consider the child's request.

The child will understand the response may be "Yes," "Yes with conditions," or "No." The child will understand that once a response is given, there will be no arguments.

_____   _____

Child's Signature   Parent's Signature

                                          _____

                                          Parent's Signature

Family contracts are great for preteens and adolescents, but may not work as well for younger children, or children with more significant needs. Being a parent can be challenging because each child may need a completely different approach to accomplish the same desired behaviors. A family contract for a twelve-year-old with autism spectrum disorder, for example, may be too lengthy and may not motivate wanted actions for where they are in development. For this child, the approach must be different. Take personal care, for instance. While an age matched neurotypical child may be expected to shower, brush their teeth, change their clothes, and care for themselves without prompting, getting a neurodiverse child to brush their teeth is a chore. Some children with sensory issues do not like the texture of the toothpaste. They may not like the sensation of the bristles of the toothbrush against their gums. This child may need prompting multiple times before the tooth brushing activity is accomplished. Many children with autism do not respond well to negative reinforcement. Telling them "If you do not brush your teeth, I will not let you watch a television show" may lead to a four-hour meltdown. Often, positive reinforcement leads to improved child compliance. Telling a child "Once your teeth are brushed, you can have thirty minutes to watch your television show" is incentive for them to keep at the activity until they have completed the task. This child may benefit at both home and school with incentive charts (sticker charts) where a completed task earned a marker on the chart, and so many markers led to a privilege or prize.

Understanding the best plan to motivate your child may not be an easy task. There are trained behavioral consultants who spend hours with an adolescent to understand what drives the individual to make certain choices they do, and then put together an analysis to help guide treatment. If your child is currently in therapy, I would involve the therapist in the family contract/behavioral plan. If your child is not currently in therapeutic services, consider a behavioral analysis through a local organization or getting the school counselor involved in assisting your efforts. Your primary care provider may also have options for developmental resources through their organization.

Homework: Prepare for your family contract (older children) or behavioral expectation chart (younger children). (Additional Matter – Preparing Your Family Contract, Behavioral Expectations for Younger Children).

Chapter 9

BREAK GLASS IN CASE OF EMERGENCY

Crisis Text Line

C risis Text Line is a 24-hour support for those in crisis. **Text 741741** from anywhere in the United States and you will receive an automated text asking you what your crisis is. Within minutes, a live crisis-trained counselor will answer your text. The text exchange is free, confidential, and will not appear on your phone statement. There is also a WhatsApp option.

Parent Resources

In my experience, mental health resources are generally passed along through word of mouth. Some of the best books, websites, treatment centers, and after care programs I have encountered were brought to my attention in conversations with behavioral health providers, physician colleagues, or patients. In this section, I have chosen those books and websites I most commonly recommend. To assist in identifying which resource may be best for you, I have added a synopsis and available formats of the material. I have no conflict of interests to disclose in resources I chose to mention. I came across many of the items I mention below I came across while trying to help my children on their mental health journey.

The following trusted mental health resources can provide you with extra support when you need it.

US National Alliance on Mental Illness (NAMI): 1-800-950-NAMI

Nationwide network and search function for support and education. https://www.nami.org/Support-Education/NAMI-HelpLine/Top-HelpLine-Resources

US National Suicide Prevention Lifeline: 1-800-273-TALK (1-800-273-8255)

Available in English, Spanish
Deaf & Hard of Hearing Options: 1-800-799-4889
https://suicidepreventionlifeline.org

US Samaritans: 1-800-870-HOPE (1-800-870-4673)

Registered charity aimed at providing emotional support to anyone in distress or at risk of suicide throughout the United States
http://www.samaritansusa.org

US SAMHSA National Helpline: 1-800-662-HELP (1-800-662-4357)

Free, confidential, 24/7, 365-day-a-year treatment referral and information service for individuals and families facing mental and/or substance use disorders
Available in English, Spanish

US Trevor Project: 1-866-488-7386

An organization that provides a 24-hour phone hotline, as well as limited-hour webchat and text options, for lesbian, gay, bisexual, transgender and questioning youth within the United States
Text TREVOR to 1-202-304-1200 (available M-F from 3:00pm to 10:00pm ET)

US Veterans Crisis Line: 1-800-273-8255

A 24/7 hotline that provides phone, webchat, and text options available to military veterans and their families.
Deaf & Hard of Hearing Options available

Recommended Apps

Calm: Sleep & Meditation

Calm has several integrative programs to help work on relaxation and emotional regulation. An individual can learn to meditate, participate in video lessons on mindful movement and gentle stretching, listen to audio programs by world-renowned mindfulness experts, and enjoy sounds of nature or soothing music throughout the course of their day.

Seller: Calm.com, Inc
Size: 105.4 MB
Age Rating: 4+
In-App Purchases: Yes

You can also access this material through their website www.calm.com

Headspace: Meditation & Sleep

Headspace was started with one mission: to improve the health and happiness of the world. Headspace has several articles, audio recordings, and lessons to teach meditation and mindfulness. Headspace is part of Headspace Health, the world's most accessible comprehensive provider of mental health and well-being care. Headspace Health also consists of Headspace for Work and Ginger, who partner with over 2,500 companies and health plans to provide access to meditation, mindfulness, coaching, therapy and psychiatry to their members and employees.

Seller: Headspace Inc.
Size: 72.8 MB
Age Rating: 4+

In-App Purchases: Yes

You can also access this material through their website www.headspace.com

MindDoc: Your Companion

MindDoc was developed by clinical psychologists in close collaboration with leading researchers for those who want to learn about emotional well-being or who suffer from mild to moderate mental illness including depression, anxiety, insomnia, and eating disorders.

Seller: MindDoc Health GmbH
Size: 17.3 MB
Age Rating: 12+
In-App Purchases: Yes

Recommended Books

An Unchanged Mind: The Problem of Immaturity in Adolescence; by John A. McKinnon MD

Synopsis: *An Unchanged Mind* tackles the question, "Why are American teenagers failing to develop normally through adolescence?" The book dives into a brief review of normal development and then examines the delays today's teenagers are suffering and the root cause behind those delays. Unfortunately, disrupted maturation leads to a flawed approach to living. Dr. McKinnon, however, leaves us with hope. With a sustained push to help troubled teenagers catch up, symptoms may improve, and academic and interpersonal skills can functionally improve.

General Length: 272 pages
Publication Date: November 30, 2008
Available Formats: ebook, Paperback

Beyond Behaviors: Using Brain Science and Compassion to Understand and Solve Children's Behavioral Challenges; by Mona Delahooke, PhD

Synopsis: In *Beyond Behaviors*, Dr. Mona Delahooke describes behaviors as the "tip of the iceberg," important signals to helping understand a child's difference in the context of relational safety. This book provides techniques to reduce behavioral challenges and promote psychological resilience while developing secure relationships. Dr. Delahooke's approach may be effective for children diagnosed with Oppositional Defiant Disorder (ODD), Conduct Disorder (CD), Disruptive Mood Dysregulation Disorder (DMDD), Anxiety & Depression, and Sensory Processing Disorder (SPD).

General Length: 317 pages

Publication Date: April 4, 2019
Available Formats: ebook, Audiobook, Paperback

Finally Focused: The Breakthrough Natural Treatment Plan for ADHD that Restores Attention, Minimizes Hyperactivity, and Helps Eliminate Drug Side Effects; by James Greenblatt MD and Bill Gottlieb CHC.

Synopsis: Dr. James Greenblatt has treated several children and adults struggling with symptoms of hyperactivity and inattention during his years as a psychiatrist. Using his effective Plus-Minus Healing Plan, parents will understand the reason behind their child's symptoms and then be able to start eliminating the unwanted behaviors by addressing the child's unique pattern of biological constituents. Dr. Greenblatt's therapeutic plan addresses more than a child's medication but uses a complementary approach to tailor remedies to individual needs.

General Length: 272 pages.
Publication Date: May 9, 2017
Available Formats: ebook, Audiobook, Paperback

Glow Kids: How Screen Addiction is Hijacking Our Kids – And How to Break the Trance; by Nicholas Kardaras, PhD

Synopsis: In *Glow Kids*, Nicholas Kardaras, PhD examines how technology, specifically, age-inappropriate screen tech, has profoundly affected the brains of an entire generation. Dr. Kardaras discusses how brain imaging research is showing that stimulating glowing screens increase dopamine in the brain's pleasure center, like how the brain experiences sexual gratification. In recent years, clinical research has found correlations between mental health conditions such as ADHD, addiction, anxiety, depression, increased aggression and even psychosis with the amount of screen time experienced by a child. This book dives into the sociological, psychological, cultural, and economic factors facing children as they grow up in a world of new technology.

General Length: 290 pages
Publication Date: August 9, 2016
Available Formats: ebook, Audiobook, Hardcover, Paperback

How to Hug a Porcupine: Negotiating the Prickly Points of the Tween Years; by Julie A. Ross, MA

Synopsis: In *How to Hug a Porcupine*, Julie A Ross, executive director of Parenting Horizons, examines the developing brain through adolescence and provides parents with the tools needed to handle this challenging time. Teenagers experience a whirlwind of changes physically and socially as they move through their middle school years. The author provides experienced solutions to helping kids learn responsibility, handle the difficulties of peer pressure, and become successful adults. She also gives tips on talking to your children about sex, drugs, and alcohol so your children will listen.

General Length: 224 pages
Publication Date: July 23, 2008
Available Formats: ebook, Audiobook, Paperback

Integrative Medicine for Binge Eating: A Comprehensive Guide to the New Hope Model for the Elimination of Binge Eating and Food Cravings; by James Greenblatt, MD

Synopsis: Dr. Greenblatt, a respected psychiatrist and eating disorder expert, explains how appetite is controlled by the brain's neurochemical systems. This book combines traditional medicine and complementary approaches for recovery from Binge Eating Disorder and food addiction. This book is based on scientific research to help individuals reclaim a health relationship with food. While not specific to children and adolescence, I found this book to be a helpful guide in understanding my child's behavior and strategies to help them develop long term success.

General Length: 300 pages
Publication Date: March 21, 2019
Available Formats: ebook, Hardcover, Paperback

Not by Chance: How Parents Boost Their Teen's Success in and After Treatment; by Tim R. Thayne, PhD

Synopsis: Dr. Tim Thayne's career has been spent working with teenagers in wilderness and residential programs. Over time, he became frustrated when adolescents who had been struggling with addictions, learning disabilities, and emotional/behavioral issues made significant progress during treatment, only to return home and have things quickly unravel. Throughout his career, Dr. Thayne's mission has become to improve long-term success in adolescents' mental health after wilderness or residential treatment. He has crafted a model to coach parents using concrete tools, backed by solid research, to help with their child's transition through treatment and back to their home environment.

General Length: 304 pages
Publication Date: April 25, 2017
Available Formats: ebook, Audiobook, Hardcover

Parenting from the Inside Out: How a Deeper Self-Understanding Can Help You Raise Children That Thrive; by Daniel J. Siegel, MD and Mary Hartzell, MEd

Synopsis: In *Parenting from the Inside Out*, child psychiatrist Dr. Daniel Siegel, and early childhood expert Mary Hartzell explore the extent our own childhood experiences affect the way we parent our offspring. The authors draw from research in neurobiology and attachment to explain how relationships between one another directly impact the developing brain. This book offers a step-by-step approach to raising compassionate and resilient children by way of understanding our own life stories.

General Length: 336 pages
Publication Date: December 26, 2013
Available Formats: ebook, Paperback

The Body Keeps the Score: Brain, Mind, and body in the Healing of Trauma; by Bessel van der Kolk, MD

Synopsis: Sadly, trauma is a fact of life. Traumatic experiences inevitably leave traces on our mind, emotions, and may even alter our biology. When an individual has suffered from a tragic event, it affects not only themselves, but also their partners and their children. Renowned trauma expert, Bessel van der Kolk, has spent over three decades working with survivors. In his book, *The Body Keeps the Score*, he transforms how we interpret traumatic stress, revealing how it alters our brain's wiring. This book helps victims reclaim their lives, even when drugs and talk therapy may have failed.

General Length: 464 pages
Publication Date: September 25, 2014
Available Formats: ebook, Audiobook, Hardcover

The Gender Identity Guide for Parents: Compassionate Advice to Help Your Child Be Their Most Authentic Self; by Tavi Hawn, LCSW.

Synopsis: Very few parents are equipped with the knowledge of how to talk to their child about gender identity. Fortunately, with the right guidance, parents may have a healthy conversation and create an affirming environment for their adolescent. Tavi Hawn, LCSW is a co-founder of QORDS, a nonprofit summer camp for queer and transgender youth and youth of LGBTQ+ families. This book helps parents learn the basics about gender identity and gender expression and discover the skills needed to maintain open communication with their child.

General Length: 156 pages
Publication Date: January 4, 2022
Available Formats: ebook, Paperback

The Parallel Process: Growing Alongside Your Adolescent or Young Adult Child in Treatment; by Krissy Pozatek, LCSW

Synopsis: For some parents of troubled teenagers, a therapeutic program that removes the child from the home for a period is needed for the family unit to succeed going forward. As difficult as it is to admit, the teenager may not be the only individual responsible for the tension that left the family under siege. A wilderness or residential treatment program may be necessary for the adolescent to embark on a journey of self-discovery, skill-development, and emotional maturation, but parents must also work on their own behaviors that may have contributed to the family's downward spiral. In The Parallel Process, adolescent and family therapist, Krissy Pozatek, helps parents understand their own behaviors, learn to attune to their emotions, and have the techniques needed to for the success of their child after treatment. I found this book to be helpful whether or not you are a parent of a troubled teen to learn skills which may be needed for navigating the teenage years with your youth.

General Length: 192 pages
Publication Date: December 1, 2010
Available Formats: ebook, Audiobook, Paperback

The Ultimate Guide to Raising Teens and Tweens: Strategies for Unlocking Your Child's Full Potential; by Douglas Haddad

Synopsis: Every parent wants what is best for their child. The teenage years come with several challenges: bullying, violence, sex, substance use, eating disorders, depression, suicide, lack of physical activity, and many more. *The Ultimate Guide to Raising Teens and Tweens* offers a step-by-step plan for raising an adolescent to be a strong and successful adult. Supported by current research, the author teaches tools to guide any family navigating the teen years.

General Length: 287 pages
Publication Date: February 16, 2017
Available Formats: ebook, Paperback

Recommended Websites

https://interface.williamjames.edu/guide/websites-especially-teens

The William James INTERFACE referral service aims to help break down the silos that exist between agencies, mental health providers, and systems that can often hinder access to wellness services for individuals. Their website offers several connections to a multitude of resources. They also offer a helpline that operates Monday to Friday to connect callers with a Resource and Referral Counselor who will help them navigate the challenges of finding an appropriate mental health service.

goaskalice.columbia.edu

Alice! is not one person, but a team. The Go Ask Alice! site is supported by a team of Columbia University health promotion specialists, health care providers, and other health professionals, along with a staff of information and research specialists and writers. Their team members have advanced degrees in public health, health education, medicine, counseling, and several other relevant fields. Go Ask Alice! is a health Q&A resource that provides readers accurate and culturally competent information so they can make responsible health and well-being decisions.

loveisrespect.org

This site is operated by the National Domestic Violence Hotline and provides access to the National Teen Dating Abuse Helpline. Teens can contact a trained peer or adult advocate anonymously and confidentially for real-time one-on-one support and information.

Resources are also available for parents, teachers, clergy, law enforcement, and health care providers.

mentalhealthliteracy.org

Canadian website that is committed to creating and delivering the highest quality mental health literacy information, research, education, and resources. Materials are provided in a variety of mediums designed to meet the needs of children, youth, young adults, families, educators, community agencies and health care providers.

teenhelp.com

TeenHelp.com was developed for teens and their parents going through common development issues. There are fact sheets, statistics, and informative guides on topics such as self-esteem, suicide, depression, trauma, substance use and developing positive relationships and moral values.

Fight the Stigma!

makeitok.org

"Make It Ok" is a campaign to reduce mental illness stigma. The campaign was made possible by several organizations that created a partnership to pledge their commitment to change the hearts and minds about the misperceptions of mental ailments by encouraging open conversation and education on the topic.

nostigmas.org

The goal of "No Stigmas" is the elimination of stigma towards mental health concerns. Their website offers free membership to anyone who agrees to uphold core values of respect, community support and advocacy for others, personal responsibility, and the elimination of stigma. Membership includes tools for awareness, information content, and access to peer groups, events, and e-learning courses. Visitors in need of support can connect online with peers, obtain information about free or low-cost counseling resources, and treatment tools.

time-to-change.org.uk

"Time to Change" is a campaign to challenge mental health stigma and discrimination. They are dedicated to making sure no one fears being treated differently because of a mental health diagnosis.

A Plea to Parents

Once upon a time, you met someone you considered to be the love of your life. The two of you shared a moment of intimacy and from that relationship came an incredible human soul. Being a parent is a very challenging feat. It means making sacrifices to help another being grow and develop to become a strong member of society. For your child to have an advantage as an adult, you've likely found yourself needing to be selfless. Perhaps you've lost sleep, given up seconds at dinner, didn't purchase that new pair of shoes, missed time at work, put your education on hold, or missed time with friends so your child could have what they needed.

Children are unable to care for themselves. Their physical and emotional needs rely heavily on the attention of their caregivers. Children belong to several types of families. Children may be raised by a biological parent, adopted parent, foster parent, or other relative. They may have one caregiver or several. Children can have one place they call home or more. They may be an only child, have siblings/half-siblings/stepsiblings/adopted siblings, or even foster siblings. Children may have full access to mental health resources or live in a location where resources are scarce.

You've likely picked up this book because your child is suffering. You've acknowledged your child needs more assistance than what you felt able to offer them. You're willing to put them first so they have the skills they need to be stronger and have a successful life. Unfortunately, not all parents feel the same way.

I have encountered various situations in my time as a parent and as a physician where the needs of the child were debated upon by those caring for the adolescent. It's sad some parents may not recognize their child needs additional resources in their development. In a handful of cultures, the stigma of mental health remains strong. For instance, 15-year-old Gabriela had been struggling with depression for a few years. Her culture views mental illness as a sign of weakness. As such, her father was very much against any treatment for her symptoms. When Gabriela stopped spending time with friends, her grades were declining, and she was losing weight from food avoidance, her mother brought her to me asking for help. Gabriela was not against therapy or medication management as she knew others that had improved with these modalities. While her mother understood Gabriela may need additional approaches for her mood, she was afraid of what her spouse may say or do. Gabriela's mother pleaded with me to prescribe her daughter medication for her mood but label it as medication to help with "menstrual cycle disorders" so Gabriela's father would not be upset. She also requested that any counseling be done at the school so Gabriela would not miss out helping at the family business after school.

Gabriela's situation was very challenging for me. On one hand, both Gabriela's mother and father a legal say in her upbringing. By starting a medication against Gabriela's father's wishes, his authoritative right to her care was being ignored. On the other hand, not starting medication was against the wishes of Gabriela and her mother, who also had input into Gabriela's upbringing. The frustration of Gabriela wanting help and seeing her father put barriers up to her getting the care she longed for ultimately strained their relationship. Gabriela no longer went to her father for assistance. She limited her social interactions with him while she completed high school. Once Gabriela moved out of the home, she maintained very little contact with her father.

Children sense when there is tension between their parents They know when parents are in a disagreement with one another on their care. Even if you have never argued in front of your child about their upbringing, trust me, they know. Disagreements felt by your offspring may increase the turmoil they feel. I understand you and others managing your child's welfare will not always see eye to eye, however, the more you can place your child's needs first and work towards the common goal of betterment for their physical and mental health the more likely your child will be to succeed. Consistency and unity, while not always easy, are important.

CONCLUSION

A ccording to the United States Center for Disease Control and Prevention, 8.9% of children ages three to 17 have been identified as having a behavioral problem (CDC, 2022). Approximately 5.8 million children, or 9.4%, children in this age group have been identified as having anxiety. Nearly three million, or 4.4%, of children have been diagnosed with depression (CDC, 2022). For many youngsters, some of these conditions commonly occur together. For instance, three in four children with depression also have anxiety and one in two children are struggling behaviorally (CDC, 2022). These numbers are shocking and are sadly growing over time. Among children ages six to 17, the rate of those "ever having been diagnosed with either anxiety or depression" grew from 5.4% in 2003 to 8.4% in 2011-2012 (CDC, 2022). Recent reports note one in six children aged two to eight years (17.4%) has been diagnosed with a mental, behavioral, or developmental disorder (CDC, 2022).

Sadly, the mental health world is one of the most challenging ones I have found to navigate. Behavioral health services may take place in a multitude of locations. The treatment facility often depends on the type and intensity of therapy that is needed. Barriers for many families seeking mental health assistance for their child include reduced number of resources available, lack of continuity between many inpatient and outpatient programs, and increased cost of treatment. Parents are often disheartened by the limited communication between the provider and themselves regarding ways to support their child during treatment. It is unfortunate many adolescents cannot get the care they require when mental health is so crucial to physical health, social relationships, work productivity, and overall psychological wellbeing.

Fortunately, there are steps parents can take to advocate for their children. Parents can encourage their child to make healthy lifestyle choices. The best way to support your child's overall wellbeing is through example. If children see their parents making wholesome choices, even under stress, they are more likely to do the same. Healthy choices include limiting technology use to two hours or less during the day, eating a balanced diet, getting adequate sleep, exercising, spending time outdoors, and connecting with the surrounding world on a spiritual level. Parents are urged to keep open communication with their child and seek individual or family counseling services when stressful situations begin to cause a significant decline in a child's wellness. If counseling appears to be ineffective alone, parents may seek out additional support through medical providers, behavioral consultants, school officials, or exploring community resources whether in-person or online.

We live in a very challenging time. Prior to the 2020 Covid 19 Pandemic, children, adolescents, and teens were struggling with mental health ailments. The pandemic aided further mental decline through increased physical illness, loss of loved ones, social isolation, and financial hardships (UNC College of Arts and Sciences, 2021). As the pandemic wore on, youth showed more consistent elevations in anxiety and depression. I believe we have yet to see the long-term effects on this generation.

You can be your child's biggest advocate for mental wellness. Even if your child is struggling now, by recognizing their need for outside help and supporting their current journey, they are more likely to become a very successful and well-adjusted adult. Most importantly, on those grey days where you feel defeated remember… YOU ARE NOT ALONE.

ADDITIONAL MATTER

(AKA... The Appendix)

For downloadable templates, visit <u>drstephaniemacke.com</u>.

Chapter 1 Homework: Your Story

(Use this space to write down your family's experience.)

_____

_____

_____

_____

_____

_____

_____

_____

_____

_____

Chapter 2 Homework: Factors Affecting Your Family's Mental Health

(Use this space to understand the genetic and environmental influences affecting your family unit. Fill in things you image fit each category, and things that overlap between factors.)

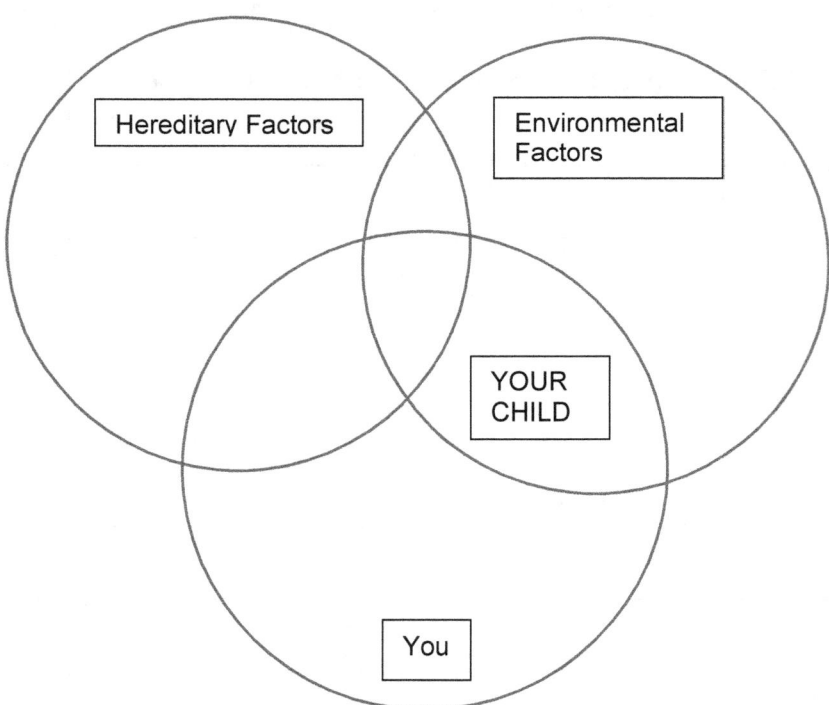

Chapter 3 Homework: Healthcare Team

Provider Name: _____ Credentials: _____

Business Name: _____

Address: _____

City: _____State: _____Zip Code: _____

Phone: (_____) _____ - _____Fax: (_____) _____ - _____

Services Provided: _____

Treating Diagnosis: _____

Medications Prescribed:

_____

_____

Provider Name: _____ Credentials: _____

Business Name: _____

Address: _____

City: _____State: _____Zip Code: _____

Phone: (_____) _____ - _____Fax: (_____) _____ - _____

Services Provided: _____

Treating Diagnosis: _____

Medications Prescribed:

_____

_____

Provider Name: _____ Credentials: _____

Business Name: _____

Address: _____

City: _____State: _____Zip Code: _____

Phone: (_____) _____ - _____Fax: (_____) _____ - _____

Services Provided: _____

Treating Diagnosis: _____

Medications Prescribed:

_____

_____

Provider Name: _____ Credentials: _____

Business Name: _____

Address: _____

City: _____State: _____Zip Code: _____

Phone: (_____) _____ - _____Fax: (_____) _____ - _____

Services Provided: _____

Treating Diagnosis: _____

Medications Prescribed:

_____

_____

Provider Name: _____ Credentials: _____

Business Name: _____

Address: _____

City: _____State: _____Zip Code: _____

Phone: (_____) _____ - _____Fax: (_____) _____ - _____

Services Provided: _____

Treating Diagnosis: _____

Medications Prescribed:

_____

_____

Provider Name: _____ Credentials: _____

Business Name: _____

Address: _____

City: _____State: _____Zip Code: _____

Phone: (_____) _____ - _____Fax: (_____) _____ - _____

Services Provided: _____

Treating Diagnosis: _____

Medications Prescribed:

_____

_____

Chapter 4 Homework: Mental Health Visit Preparation

Name: _____ DOB: _____/_____/_____

Past medical history (Illnesses, Previous Diagnoses):

_____

_____

Past hospitalizations (Include Dates if Possible):

_____

_____

Past surgical history:_____
Current medications (Include Vitamins, Supplements, Herbs in
addition to Prescriptions):_____

_____

_____

Allergies:_____
Social history:
    Who lives in the home?_____
    What school does the child attend? _____
    Does the child smoke? _____
    Does the child use alcohol? _____
    Does the child use illegal substances? _____
Sexual history:
    Is the child sexually active?_____
    What gender does the child identify with? _____
Family History:
    Mother: _____
    Father: _____
    Brother: _____
    Sister: _____
    Maternal grandmother: _____
    Maternal grandfather: _____
    Paternal grandfather: _____
    Paternal grandmother:_____

Immunization history: Are the child's immunizations up to date? _____

Current health care professionals: (Please include Primary Care, Counselors, Psychologists, Psychiatrists, etc. Include addresses and phone numbers if possible).

_____

_____

_____

_____

_____

CC: _____

Recent events:

_____

_____

_____

What was/were the precipitating factor(s)?

_____

_____

What is the extent of the condition?

_____

What are the primary symptoms?

_____

_____

What is the duration of the symptoms?

_____

Has the child ever had any concerns like this previously?

_____

Has the child mentioned thoughts of harming themselves or someone else?

_____

Itinerary (Things to Discuss):

1. _____
2. _____
3. _____

Medication Refills Needed (Name of Medication, Dose, and Frequency):

_____

_____

_____

_____

_____

_____

_____

_____

_____

_____

_____

_____

Chapter 5 Homework: Your Child's Characteristics

Has your child been diagnosed with a particular condition? If so, use this space to write down the diagnosis, name of the provider who assessed your child, and date of the assessment. This information will be valuable in future treatment planning. If your child has not had an assessment, has not yet been diagnosed with a particular mental health condition, use this space to write down characteristics you have observed that you want to remember to bring up with your child's healthcare provider.

_____

_____

_____

_____

_____

_____

_____

_____

_____

_____

_____

_____

_____

_____

_____

_____

Chapter 6 Homework: Learn and Practice Emotional Regulation Techniques

Emotion regulation is the process of controlling one's emotions, keeping them in balance and away from extremes. Below are some skills to teach your child to help calm their "irrational brain" when it's in overdrive. Please note, these skills can be helpful in a moment of crisis, but generally will not be effective if taught during the time of distress. A marathon runner would not wake up one sunny morning and say, "I think I'll run 26 miles today!" after not having ever exercised. The athlete would train, and practice, and gradually build up their endurance to accomplish such a feat. Similarly, emotional regulation techniques should be taught, practiced, and then utilized during heightened emotional states.

Box Breathing

U.S. Navy SEALs work under high-stress situations. To aid in stress management and overall wellness, Navy SEALs use a technique known as box breathing (MedicineNet, 2021). To perform this technique:

a. Slowly exhale to the count of four.

b. Hold your breath to the count of four.

c. Breathe in to the count of four.

d. Hold your breath to the count of four.

e. Repeat.

5-4-3-2-1 Grounding Technique

The goal of this exercise is to use the five senses to focus on the moment and avoid multiple anxious thoughts that can get in your way of progress.

a. What are five things that you can see?

b. What are four things that you can feel?

c. What are three things that you can hear?

d. What are two things that you can smell?

e. What is one thing that you can taste?

4 Line Feelings Check

If I'm journaling, I find this is a great way to start. This helps me reflect on where I am in the moment.

a. Body – How do you feel physically? (Relaxed, Tense, Fatigued, etc.)

b. Mind – How do you feel mentally? (Busy, Calm, etc.)

c. Heart – How do you feel emotionally? (Happy, Frustrated, Disheartened, etc.)

d. Soul – How do you feel spiritually? (Connected, isolated, etc.)

STOPP

STOPP is a strategy that will help you in the heat of the moment. It incorporates aspects of CBT, DBT and mindfulness meditation.

a. S – Stop!

Pause for a moment.

b. T – Take a breath.

Notice your breathing as you inhale and then exhale.

c. O – Observe.

What thoughts are racing through your mind?

What are you responding to?

What sensations do you feel physically in your body?

d. P – Pull Back.

What is the bigger picture?

Is this thought a fact or an opinion?

How important is this? Will this matter several months from now?

e. P – Proceed.

What is the best thing to do right now?

Do what will be effective and appropriate.

Practice Makes Perfect

It takes a good 21 days for a new habit to become a routine. Make a commitment with your child to practice an emotional regulation skill every day for 21 days. Perhaps entice them with positive reinforcement. For instance, seven days of practice allows them to stay up for an extra hour. Maybe 14 days of practice allows them to have a friend spend the night. If the skills are performed for 21 days in a row, they earn an outing. Be creative with what works or your family. Choose rewards that motivate your child.

Day #	Skill Practiced	Day #	Skill Practiced
1	_____	11	_____
2	_____	12	_____
3	_____	13	_____
4	_____	14	_____
5	_____	15	_____
6	_____	16	_____
7	_____	17	_____
8	_____	18	_____
9	_____	19	_____
10	_____	20	_____
		21	_____

Homework Chapter 7: Medication Management

Pharmacy: _____

Address: _____

Phone: (_____) _____-_____

Medication Name/Dose: _____

Time of Day Taken:_____AM_____Mid_____PM

Start Date: _____/_____/_____

Prescriber: _____

Side Effects: _____

Stop Date: _____/_____/_____

Medication Name/Dose:_____

Time of Day Taken:_____AM_____Mid_____PM

Start Date: _____/_____/_____

Prescriber: _____

Side Effects: _____

Stop Date: _____/_____/_____

Medication Name/Dose: _____

Time of Day Taken:_____AM_____Mid_____PM

Start Date: _____/_____/_____

Prescriber: _____

Side Effects: _____

Stop Date: _____/_____/_____

Medication Name/Dose: _____

Time of Day Taken:_____AM_____Mid_____PM

Start Date: _____/_____/_____

Prescriber: _____

Side Effects: _____

Stop Date: _____/_____/_____

Medication Name/Dose: _____

Time of Day Taken:_____AM_____Mid_____PM

Start Date: _____/_____/_____

Prescriber: _____

Side Effects: _____

Stop Date: _____/_____/_____

Medication Name/Dose: _____

Time of Day Taken:_____AM_____Mid_____PM

Start Date: _____/_____/_____

Prescriber: _____

Side Effects: _____

Stop Date: _____/_____/_____

Medication Name/Dose: _____

Time of Day Taken:_____AM_____Mid_____PM

Start Date: _____/_____/_____

Prescriber: _____

Side Effects: _____

Stop Date: _____/_____/_____

Medication Name/Dose: _____

Time of Day Taken:_____AM_____Mid_____PM

Start Date: _____/_____/_____

Prescriber: _____

Side Effects: _____

Stop Date: _____/_____/_____

Homework Chapter 8: Preparing Your Family Contract

Our family mission: (What does your family value? How do you want to be sure those values are carried out by family members?)

_____

_____

Family Relationships
(What are the expectations for being a member of the family?)

1. _____

2. _____

3. _____

4. _____

5. _____

Consequences of respectful behavior include:

1. _____

2. _____

3. _____

4. _____

5. _____

Consequences of disrespectful behavior include:

1. _____

2. _____

3. _____

4. _____

5. _____

Personal Care
(What are the expectations for self-care?)

1. _____
2. _____
3. _____
4. _____
5. _____

Consequences for maintaining personal include:

1. _____
2. _____
3. _____
4. _____
5. _____

Consequences for not maintaining personal care include:

1. _____
2. _____
3. _____
4. _____
5. _____

School
(What are the educational expectations for the child?)

1. _____
2. _____
3. _____
4. _____
5. _____

Consequences when schoolwork is managed:

1. _____
2. _____
3. _____
4. _____
5. _____

Consequences when schoolwork is not managed:

1. _____
2. _____
3. _____
4. _____
5. _____

Cell Phone and Electronic Devices
(What are the expectations for managing technology?)

1. _____
2. _____
3. _____
4. _____
5. _____

Consequences from following electronic guidelines:

1. _____
2. _____
3. _____
4. _____
5. _____

Consequences from not following electronic guidelines:

1. _____
2. _____
3. _____
4. _____
5. _____

Friends
(What are the expectations for time with friends?)

1. _____
2. _____
3. _____
4. _____
5. _____

Consequences for following friend guidelines:

1. _____
2. _____
3. _____
4. _____
5. _____

Consequences for not following friend guidelines:

1. _____
2. _____
3. _____
4. _____
5. _____

Curfew
(What are the expectations for returning home?)

1. _____
2. _____
3. _____
4. _____
5. _____

Consequences for following curfew guidelines:

1. _____
2. _____
3. _____
4. _____
5. _____

Consequences for not following curfew guidelines:

1. _____
2. _____
3. _____
4. _____
5. _____

Driving
(What are the expectations for operating a vehicle?)

1. _____
2. _____
3. _____
4. _____
5. _____

Consequences for following driving guidelines:

1. _____
2. _____
3. _____
4. _____
5. _____

Consequences for not following driving guidelines:

1. _____
2. _____
3. _____
4. _____
5. _____

Requesting to Make Changes to the
Family Contract

A child may make a request to the parent(s) to addend the Family Contract. Before submitting the request, the child:

1. Will take the time to consider what concerns the parents may have with the request.

2. Be ready to suggest solutions to resolve parent concerns.

3. Given enough time for the child and the parent(s) to discuss the requested change.

The parent(s) will take time to consider the child's request.

The child will understand the response may be "Yes," "Yes with conditions," or "No." The child will understand that once a response is given, there will be no arguments.

_____   _____

Child's Signature   Parent's Signature

                                                            _____

                                                            Parent's Signature

Behavioral Expectations for Younger Children

	Monday	Tuesday	Wednesday	Thursday	Friday	Saturday	Sunday
Brush Teeth							
Shower							
Put on Clean Clothes							
Complete Homework							
Clean Bedroom							
Brush Dog							
Vacuum Room							
Take Out Trash							

*The above table represents an example of a check off table to earn privileges or rewards.

REFERENCES

Acceptance and Commitment Therapy. (2022). *CBT Associates*. Retrieved from https://www.cbtassociates.com/about-us/the-cbt-approach/#mindfulness.

Ackerman, C. (2017). How Does Acceptance and Commitment Therapy (ACT) Work?

Positive Psychology. Retrieved from https://positivepsychology.com/act-acceptance-and-commitment-therapy/.

Adikwu, M. (2020). What is CPT Therapy and How Does It Help PTSD? *TalkSpace*. Retrieved from https://www.talkspace.com/blog/cpt-cognitive-processing-therapy-what-is-definition-get-started-guide/.

Alcohol Abuse Statistics. (2022). *National Center for Drug Abuse Statistics*. Retrieved from https://drugabusestatistics.org/alcohol-abuse-statistics/.

Agutter P.S., & Wheatley D.N. (2007). *Stability and Change in DNA. In: About Life*. Springer, Dordrecht. Retrieved from https://doi.org/10.1007/978-1-4020-5418-1_11.

American Psychiatric Association. (2013). Diagnostic and Statistical manual of Mental Disorders. 5th ed. Washington, DC: American Psychiatric Association.

Arain M., Haque M., Johal L., Mathur P., Nel W., Rais A., Sandhu R., & Sharma S. (2013). Maturation of the adolescent brain. *Neuropsychiatric Disease and Treatment*. 9, 449-461.

Ardito, A. (2020). What is an LCSW? *Choosing Therapy*. Retrieved from https://www.choosingtherapy.com/what-is-an-lcsw/.

Berzin, R. (2018). 8 Causes Behind Your Anxiety and Depression. *Parsley Health*. Retrieved from https://www.parsleyhealth.com/blog/8-causes-behind-fatigue-anxiety-depression/.

Bratten, E.B. (2011). *How to Find Mental Health Care for Your Child*. Washington, DC: American Psychological Association.

Chang J.G., Cimino F.M., & Gossa W. (2020). ADHD in Children: Common Questions and Answers. *American Family Physician*. 102(10), 592-602A.

Chapman, A.L. (2006). Dialectical Behavior Therapy: Current Indications and Unique Elements. *Psychiatry*. 3(9), 62-68.

Charles S. (2022). 5 Mental Benefits of Exercise. *Walden University*. Retrieved from https://www.waldenu.edu/online-bachelors-programs/bs-in-psychology/resource/five-mental-benefits-of-exercise.

Chevalier G., Sinatra S.T., Oschman J.L., Sokal K., & Sokal, P. (2012) Health Implications of Reconnecting the Human Body to the Earth's Surface Electrons. *Journal of Environmental Public Health*. 2012, 291541.

Coffey S.F., Banducci A.N., & Vinci C. (2015). Common Questions about Cognitive Behavior Therapy for Psychiatric Disorders. *American Family Physician*. 92(9), 807-812.

Cognitive Processing Therapy for PTSD. (2022). *U.S. Department of Veterans Affairs. National Center for PTSD*. Retrieved from https://www.ptsd.va.gov/understand_tx/cognitive_processing.asp.

Contents of the IEP. (2022). *Center for Parent Information & Resources*. Retrieved from https://www.parentcenterhub.org/iepcontents/.

Cuncic, A. (2022). How Can GABA Be Used for Social Anxiety. *Verywell Mind*. Retrieved from https://www.verywellmind.com/what-is-gaba-3024566.

Data and Statistics on Children's Mental Health. (2022). *Centers for Disease Control and Prevention*. Retrieved from https://www.cdc.gov/childrensmentalhealth/data.html.Davalon, B.Y. (2022). Understanding a Health Insurance Copayment. *eHealth*. Retrieved from https://www.ehealthinsurance.com/resources/small-business/understanding-health-insurance-copayment

Depression and Bipolar Disorder Increase Heart Disease Risk in Teens. (2022). *CardioSmart: American College of Cardiology.* Retrieved from https://www.cardiosmart org/news/2015/9/depression-and-bipolar-disorder-increase-heart-disease-risk-in-teens#:~:text=Finally%2C%20research%20suggests%20that%20depression,together%20to%20increase%20cardiovascular%20risk

Devlin, K. (2022). How Much Does a Psychologist Cost, And Is It Worth It? *ReGain Editorial Team.* Retrieved from https://www.regain.us/advice/psychology/how-much-does-a-psychologist-cost-and is-it-worth-it/.

Diagnosis. (2022). *Google.* Retrieved from https://www.google.com/search?q=diagnosis+definition&rlz=1C5CHFA_enUS967J S968&oq=diagnosis+defin&aqs=chrome.0.0i433i512j69i57j0i512l8.2055j1j15&sourc eid=chrome&ie=UTF-8.

Effects of Technology on Children During a Pandemic. (2021). *Regis College.* Retrieved from https://online.regiscollege.edu/blog/effects-of-technology-on-children/.

Elia, J. (2021). Depressive Disorders in Children and Adolescents. *Merck Manual Profession Version.* Retrieved from https://www.merckmanuals.com/professional/pediatrics/mental-disorders-in-children-and-adolescents/depressive-disorders-in-children-and-adolescents.

Eye Movement Desensitization and Reprocessing Therapy. (2022). *Indiana Health Group.* Retrieved from https://www.indianahealthgroup.com/services/emdr/.

Fabiani, A. (2021). 10 cultures that have accepted non-binary gender identities for centuries. *Screenshot.* Retrieved from https://screenshot-media.com/politics/lgbtqi-rights/non-binary-cultures/.

Fenske J.N, & Petersen K. (2013). Obsessive-Compulsive Disorder: Diagnosis and Management. *American Family Physician.* 92(10), 896-903.

Fabry, M. (2016). Now You Know: Which Came First, the Chicken or the Egg? *Time.* Retrieved from https://time.com/4475048/which-came-first-chicken-egg/.

Farber N.B., & Olney J.W. (2003). Drugs of Abuse that Cause Developing Neurons to Commit Suicide. *Developmental Brain Research.* 147(1-2), 37-45.

Fazio, C. (2021) How Much Does Primary Care Cost? *South Pointe Healthcare.* Retrieved from https://southpointehealthcare.com/primary-care/how-much-does-primary-care-cost/.

Find a Psychiatrist. *American Psychiatric Association.* Retrieved from https://finder.psychiatry.org/.

Frequently Asked Questions on Patents and Exclusivity. (2020). *U.S. Food and Drug Administration.* Retrieved from https://www.fda.gov/drugs/development-approval-process-drugs/frequently-asked-questions-patents-and-exclusivity#:~:text=Currently%2C%20the%20term%20of%20a,filed%20in%20the%20United%20States.

Glade, M.J., & Smith, K. (2015) Phosphatidylserine and the human brain. *Nutrition.* 31(6), 781-786.

Greenblatt J, & Gottlieb B. (2017). *Finally Focused: The Breakthrough Natural Treatment Plan for ADHD that Restores Attention, Minimizes Hyperactivity, and Helps Eliminate Drug Side Effects.* New York, NY: Harmony Books.

Greenblatt J, & Lee W. (2019). *Integrative Medicine for Depression: A Breakthrough Treatment Plan that Eliminates Depression Naturally.* Victoria, BC: Friesen Press.

Greenblatt J, & Ross-Taylor, V. (2019). *Integrative Medicine for Binge Eating: A comprehensive guide to the New Hope Model for the elimination of binge eating and food cravings.* Victoria, BC: Friesen Press.

Gupta P., Tiwari S., & Haria J. (2014). Relationship Between Depression and Vitamin C Status: A Study on Rural Patients from Western Uttar Pradesh in India. *International Journal of Scientific Study.* (1)4, 37-39.

Hendriksen, E. (2019). Failure to Launch Syndrome. *Scientific American.* https://www.scientificamerican.com/article/failure-to-launch-syndrome/#:~:text=Call%20it%20failure%20to%20launch,Hendriksen%20on%20May%2018%2C%202019.

Hirschfeld R., Williams J., & Spitzer R.L., et al. (2000). Development and Validation of a Screening Instrument for Bipolar Spectrum Disorder: The Mood Disorder Questionnaire. *Am J Psychiatry.* 157, 1873-1875.

Hofmeister S., & Bodden S. (2016). Premenstrual Syndrome and Premenstrual Dysphoric Disorder. *American Family Physician.* 94(3), 236-240.

How it works – Cognitive Behavioral Therapy (CBT). (2019). NHS. Retrieved from https://www.nhs.uk/mental-health/talking-therapies-medicine-treatments/talking-therapies-and-counselling/cognitive-behavioural-therapy-cbt/how-it-works/#:~:text=If%20you%20have%20CBT%20on,anxiety%20reduces%20during%20the%20session.

How Much Do Therapeutic Boarding Schools Cost? (2022). *The Envoy Group.* Retrieved from https://www.theenvoygroup.com/parents/therapeutic-boarding-school-cost/.

How to Pay for Therapeutic Boarding Schools, Residential Treatment Centers, and Wilderness Therapy Programs. (2022). *The Envoy Group.* Retrieved from https://www.theenvoygroup.com/pay-therapeutic-boarding-schools-residential-treatment-centers-wilderness-therapy-programs/.

Intensive Outpatient Programs (IOP): What Is It & Find IOPs Near Me. (2022). *American Addiction Centers.* Retrieved from https://americanaddictioncenters.org/intensive-outpatient-programs

Intimate Partner Violence. (2012, 2022). *ACOG.* Retrieved from https://www.acog.org/clinical/clinical-guidance/committee-opinion/articles/2012/02/intimate-partner-violence.

Kane L. (2021). Death by 1000 Cuts: Medscape National Physician Burnout and Suicide Report 2021. *Medscape.* Retrieved from https://www.medscape.com/slideshow/2021-lifestyle-burnout-6013456?faf=1.

Kardaras N. (2016). *Glow Kids.* New York, NY: St Martin's Press.

Kava Kava. (2022). *Mount Sinai.* Retrieved from https://www.mountsinai.org/health-library/herb/kava-kava#:~:text=In%20addition%20to%20its%20ceremonial,insomnia%2C%20and%20related%20nervous%20disorders.

Klein D.A., Paradise S.L., & Goodwin E.T. (2018). Caring for Transgender and Gender-Diverse Persons: What Clinicians Should Know. *American Family Physician.* 98(11), 645-653A.

Klein D.A., Sylvester J.E., & Schvey N.A. (2021). Eating Disorders in Primary Care: Diagnosis and Management. *American Family Physician.* 103(1), 22-34.

Krans B. (2013). Study: Depression During Pregnancy Increases a Child's Risk of Mood Disorders. *Healthline*. Retrieved from https://www.healthline.com/health-news/women-depression-during-pregnancy-increases-childs-risk-of-mood-disorders-100913.

Kubala, J. (2021). 11 Herbs and Supplements to Help Fight Depression. *Healthline*. Retrieved from https://www.healthline.com/nutrition/herbs-supplements-for-depression.

Kundakovic M., & Champagne F.A. (2015). Early-Life Experiences, Epigenetics, and the Developing Brain. *Neuropsychopharmacology*. 40, 141-153.

Kunst J. (2014). What's the Couch Got to do With It? *Psychology Today*. Retrieved from https://www.psychologytoday.com/us/blog/headshrinkers-guide-the-galaxy/201404/whats-the-couch-got-do-it.

Lillig M. (2018). Conduct Disorder: Recognition and Management. *American Family Physician*. 98(10), 585-592A.

Lightner, L. (2022). When Should the School Respond to IEP Requests or Evals? *A Day In Our Shoes*. Retrieved from https://adayinourshoes.com/iep-timeline-how-long-does-the-school-have-to/.

Locke A.B., Kirst N., & Shultz C.G. (2015). Diagnosis and Management of Generalized Anxiety Disorder and Panic Disorder in Adults. *American Family Physician*. 91(9), 617-624.

Machova K., Prochazkova R., Riha M., & Svobodova I. (2019). The Effect of Animal-Assisted Therapy on the State of Patients' Health After a Stroke: A Pilot Study. *International Journal of Environmental Research and Public Health*. 16, 3272.

Marcus D.A., Bernstein C.D., Constantin J.M., Kunkel F.A., Breuer P., & Hanlon R.B. (2012). Animal-Assisted Therapy at an Outpatient Pain Management Clinic. *Pain Medicine*. 13, 45-47.

Marcus D.A., Bernstein C.D., Constantin J.M., Kunkel F.A., Breuer P., & Hanlon R.B. (2013) Impact of Animal-Assisted Therapy for Outpatients with Fibromyalgia. *Pain Med*. 14(1), 43-51.

Marzani G., & Neff A.P. (2021). Bipolar Disorders: Evaluation and Treatment. *American Family Physician*. 103(4), 227-239.

Maurer D.M., Raymond T.J., & Davis B.N (2018). Depression: Screening and Diagnosis. *American Family Physician.* 98(8), 508-515.

Meditation Can Change Your Brain and Your Genes. (2018). *Health & Wellness.* Retrieved from https://www.communitymedical.org/about-us/news/meditation-can-change-your-brain-and-your-genes.

Mental Health Benefits of Being Outdoors. (2020). *Lifeworks.* Retrieved from https://lifeworkscc.com/mental-health-benefits-outdoors/.

Nagata J.M., Cortez C.A., Cattle C.J., & et al. (2022). Screen Time Use Among US Adolescents During the Covid-19 Pandemic: Findings From the Adolescent Brain Cognitive Development (ABCD) Study. *JAMA Pediatr.* 176(1), 94-96.
NAMI HelpLine. *National Alliance on Mental Illness.* Retrieved from https://www.nami.org/help.

Peterson, A.L. (2019). *Psych Meds Made Simple: How & Why They Do What They Do.* Mental Health @ Home Books.

Premenstrual Dysphoric Disorder (PMDD). (2022). *Johns Hopkins Medicine.* Retrieved from https://www.hopkinsmedicine.org/health/conditions-and-diseases/premenstrual-dysphoric-disorder-pmdd.

Protecting Students with Disabilities. (2020). *U.S. Department of Education Office of Civil Rights.* Retrieved from https://www2.ed.gov/about/offices/list/ocr/504faq.html#:~:text=To%20be%20protected%20under%20Section,as%20having%20such%20an%20impairment.

Psychologists. (2022). *U.S. Bureau of Labor Statistics.* Retrieved from https://www.bls.gov/ooh/life-physical-and-social-science/psychologists.htm.

Purse, M. (2022). Extrapyramidal Side Effects from Medication. *Verywell Mind.* Retrieved from https://www.verywellmind.com/extrapyramidal-side-effects-380021#:~:text=Extrapyramidal%20side%20effects%20are%20a,muscles%2C%20and%20involuntary%20facial%20movements.

Rafferty, J. (2022). Gender Identity Development in Children. Healthy Children.Org. Retrieved from https://www.healthychildren.org/English/ages-stages/gradeschool/Pages/Gender-Identity-and-Gender-Confusion-In-Children.aspx.

Rice, M. (2021). How Much Does a Psychiatrist Cost without Insurance? *Talkspace.* Retrieved from https://www.talkspace.com/blog/how-much-does-a-psychiatrist-cost/#:~:text=According%20to%20Electronic%20Health%20Reporter,your%20care%20and%20therapy%20session.

Riley M., Ahmed S., & Locke A. (2016) Common Questions About Oppositional Defiant Disorder. *American Family Physician.* 93(7), 586-591.

Schimelpfening, N (2020). 10 Drugs That Can Cause Depression. *Very Well Mind.* Retrieved from https://www.verywellmind.com/drugs-that-can-cause-depression-1067458.

Schimelpfening, N. (2021). What is Dialectical Behavioral Therapy (DBT)? *Very Well Mind.* Retrieved from https://www.verywellmind.com/dialectical-behavior-therapy-1067402.

Schmidt, J. (2022) Understanding the Differences between an IEP and a 504 Plan. *N2Y.* Retrieved from https://www.n2y.com/blog/iep-vs-504-plan/.

Scott, A. (2003). *Aristotle's Metaphysics.* Retrieved from https://www.angelfire.com/md2/timewarp/firstphilosophy.html.

Seasonal affective disorder treatment: Choosing a light box. (2022). Mayo Clinic. Retrieved from https://www.mayoclinic.org/diseases-conditions/seasonal-affective-disorder/in-depth/seasonal-affective-disorder-treatment/art-20048298.

Serotonin Syndrome. (2022). Mayo Clinic. Retrieved from https://www.mayoclinic.org/diseases-conditions/serotonin-syndrome/symptoms-causes/syc-20354758.

Sexual Violence is Preventable. (2022). *Centers for Disease Control and Prevention.* Retrieved from https://www.cdc.gov/injury/features/sexual-violence/index.html.

Sleep Hygiene Tips. (2022). *American Sleep Association.* Retrieved from https://www.sleepassociation.org/about-sleep/sleep-hygiene-tips/.

Sleep in Middle and High School Students. (2020). *Centers for Disease Control and Prevention.* Retrieved from https://www.cdc.gov/healthyschools/features/students-sleep.htm#:~:text=Importance%20of%20Sleep&text=The%20American%20Academy%20of%20Sleep,10%20hours%20per%2024%20hours.

Smith, A. (2021). What is Major Depression With Anxious Distress? Part 3: Identifying and understanding major depression subtypes. *Psychology Today.* Retrieved from https://www.psychologytoday.com/us/blog/and-running/202110/what-is-major-depression-anxious-distress.

Smith, C. (2015). Anatomy and Physiology: The Limbic System's Major Three. *Visible Body.* Retrieved from: https://www.visiblebody.com/blog/anatomy-physiology-limbic- system.

Stoppler, M.C. (2021). Definition of Filler. *RxList.* Retrieved from https://www.rxlist.com/filler/definition.htm.

Thayne, T.R. (2013). *Not By Chance.* Charleston, SC: Advantage. ebook.

The brain consumes half of a child's energy - and that could matter for weight gain: New paper proposes that variation in brain energy expenditure during childhood could be linked to obesity risk. (2019). *ScienceDaily.* Retrieved from www.sciencedaily.com/releases/2019/06/190617164629.htm.

The Four Stages of Dialectical Behavior. (2022). *Delray Center for Healing.* Retrieved from https://www.delraycenter.com/the-four-stages-of-dialectical-behavior-therapy/.

The Impact of Covid-19 on adolescents' mental health. (2021). *UNC College of Arts and Sciences.* Retrieved from https://college.unc.edu/2021/11/covid-mental-health/

The Mind and Mental Health: How Stress Affects the Brain. (2016). *Touro University Worldwide.* Retrieved from https://www.tuw.edu/health/how-stress-affects-the-brain/.

Thomas, S. (2021). The Cost to Attend an IOP. *American Addiction Centers.* Retrieved from https://americanaddictioncenters.org/intensive-outpatient-programs/cost.

Turban, J. (2020). What is Gender Dysphoria? *American Psychiatric Association.* Retrieved from https://psychiatry.org/patients-families/gender-dysphoria/what-is-gender-dysphoria.

Ultimate Guide: Independent Educational Consultant. (2022). *College Planner Pro.* Retrieved from https://www.collegeplannerpro.com/independent-educational-consultants#:~:text=Independent%20educational%20consultant%20fees%20are,includes%20and%20the%20consultant's%20experience.

Van der Kolk, B. (2014). *The Body Keeps Score: Brain, Mind, and Body in the Healing of Trauma.* New York, NY: Penguin Books.

Warner C.H., Warner C.M., Appenzeller, G.N., & Hoge, C.W. (2013). Identifying and Managing Posttraumatic Stress Disorder. *American Family Physician.* 88(12), 827-834.

What is an employee assistance program (EAP)? (2022). *United States Office of Personal Management (OPM).* Retrieved from https://www.opm.gov/faqs/QA.aspx?fid=4313c618-a96e-4c8e-b078-1f76912a10d9&pid=2c2b1e5b-6ff1-4940-b478-34039a1e1174#:~:text=Search%20by%20keywords%3A-,What%20is%20an%20Employee%20Assistance%20Program%20(EAP)%3F,%2For%20work%2Drelated%20problems.

What is a Gene? (2021). *Medline Plus.* Retrieved from https://medlineplus.gov/genetics/understanding/basics/gene/#:~:text=In%20humans%2C%20genes%20vary%20in,between%2020%2C000%20and%2025%2C000%20genes.

What is an employee assistance program (EAP)? (2022). *SHRM.* Retrieved from https://www.shrm.org/resourcesandtools/tools-and-samples/hr-qa/pages/whatisaneap.aspx.

What is Cognitive Behavioral Therapy? (2017). *PTSD Clinical Practice Guideline.* Retrieved from https://www.apa.org/ptsd-guideline/patients-and-families/cognitive-behavioral.

What is EMDR? (2020). *EMDR Institute, Inc.* Retrieved from https://www.emdr.com/what-is-emdr/.

What is Exposure Therapy? (2017). *Clinical Practice Guideline for the Treatment of PTSD.* Retrieved from https://www.apa.org/ptsd-guideline/patients-and-families/exposure-therapy#:~:text=Exposure%20therapy%20is%20a%20psychological,feared%20objects%2C%20activities%20or%20situations.

What is MBSR? (2022). *Institute for Mindfulness-Based Approaches.* Retrieved from https://www.institute-for-mindfulness.org/offer/mbsr/what-is-mbsr.

What is Solutions Focused Therapy? (2022). *Institute for Solution-Focused Therapy*. Retrieved from https://solutionfocused.net/what-is-solution-focused-therapy/.

What is the Average Fee for a Mental Health Consultant? (2022). *BikeHike*. Retrieved from https://bikehike.org/what-is-the-average-fee-for-an-mental-health-consultant/.

What is the Difference Between an IEP and a 504 Plan? (2022). *Disabilities, Opportunities, Internetworking, and Technology*. Retrieved from https://www.washington.edu/doit/what-difference-between-iep-and-504-plan#:~:text=The%20504%20Plan%20is%20a,access%20to%20the%20learning%20environment.

What to Expect. (2021). When Does Your Baby Develop a Brain? Retrieved from https://www.whattoexpect.com/pregnancy/fetal-development/fetal-brain-nervous-system/.

Wilkes, J. (2018). Gender-Dysphoric/Gender-Incongruent Persons: Treatment Recommendations from the Endocrine Society. *American Family Physicians*. 97(9), 608-609.

Why do Navy SEALs Use Box Breathing? (2021). *MedicineNet*. Retrieved from https://www.medicinenet.com/why_do_navy_seals_use_box_breathing/article.htm.

Wilder, J. (2017). How Much Does Wilderness Therapy Cost. *All Kinds of Therapy*. Retrieved from https://www.allkindsoftherapy.com/blog/how-much-does-wilderness-therapy-cost.

Wu, B. (2016). Can L-Theanine Help Treat Symptoms of Bipolar Disorder? *Healthline*. Retrieved from https://www.healthline.com/health/bipolar-disorder/l-theanine#:~:text=L%2Dtheanine%20is%20a%20relaxing,the%20dry%20weight%20of%20tea.

Your Brain on Omega-3 Fatty Acids. (2020). *The Better Fish*. Retrieved from https://www.thebetterfish.com/thecurrent/omega-3s-and-brain-health/.

ABOUT THE AUTHOR

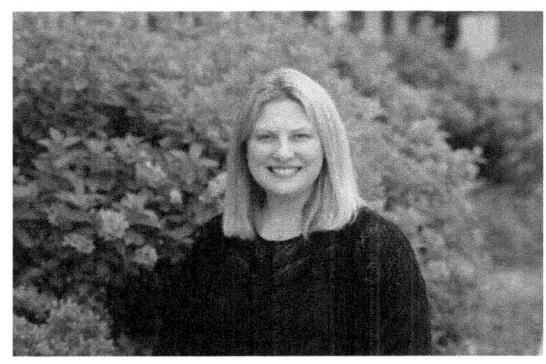

A skilled family physician, Dr. Stephanie Macke practices medicine in Speedway, Indiana. Dr. Macke believes in a holistic approach to caring for her patients and routinely evaluates the patient's physiological, psychological, social, and spiritual health. Her practice style incorporates integrative approaches to medicine. To help patients achieve optimal well-being, she utilizes various supplementations, acupuncture, manual treatments, and animal therapy in addition to traditional medicine.

Dr. Macke attended Michigan State University in East Lansing, Michigan, where she earned her Doctor of Osteopathic Medicine degree. After college, she selected Indianapolis to complete her residency at Westview Hospital and was a co-chief resident of her Family Medicine program. In pursuit of clinical excellence, Dr. Macke became board certified by the American Osteopathic Board of Family Medicine (AOBFM) and completed certification in acupuncture through Helms Medical Institute. She was featured in Top Doctors in 2019, 2021, and 2022.

Dr. Macke is loyal to the osteopathic philosophy of care and passionate about outreach initiatives that improve the health and wellness of the community. She currently serves on several hospital committees for quality and primary care redesign. She is listed as a Clinical Assistant Professor at Marian University College of Osteopathic Medicine. She has participated in global outreach programs to El Salvador, Guatemala, and India. She also served on the Board of Trustees for the Indiana Osteopathic Association from May 2011 until December 2019 and currently brings an osteopathic perspective as chairman of her network's board of directors.

Dr. Macke is married to Steven Macke and together they raise five children and two dogs. She enjoys traveling, reading, and gardening. She is at peace when she can connect to nature, likes conversations with her spouse on the back porch in the summer evenings, and always welcomes a good cup of coffee. Dr. Macke is passionate about mental health.

For additional information and up-to-date content, visit
drstephaniemacke.com.

www.ingramcontent.com/pod-product-compliance
Lightning Source LLC
Chambersburg PA
CBHW060251150626
46553CB00019BA/1585